Health Informatics

Sajeesh Kumar
Editor

Teledentistry

Springer

Editor
Sajeesh Kumar, PhD
Department of Health Informatics
University of Tennessee
Health Science Center
Memphis, TN
USA

ISBN 978-3-319-35407-1 ISBN 978-3-319-08973-7 (eBook)
DOI 10.1007/978-3-319-08973-7
Springer Cham Heidelberg New York Dordrecht London

Printed on acid-free paper

Springer is part of Springer Science+Business Media (www.springer.com)

Preface

This first-ever book on teledentistry is presented in a way that should make it accessible to anyone, independent of their knowledge of technology. This book is designed to be used by all, including clinicians, nurses, allied health professionals, and students.

The import of communication and digital technology into the field of dentistry has opened new vistas in patient care, distance learning for dental personnel, and dental care education for patients. Teledentistry is a means of achieving equity in specialist dental service delivery with acceptable levels of care that is evidence based even in situations where trained specialist personnel and infrastructure resources are limited. This multiauthor sourcebook is a collection of articles from a range of countries that not only describe what is already available but also postulate what the future holds for teledentistry.

The exciting and rapidly developing field of teledentistry encompasses high-resolution digital imaging, image storage and transmission to expert disease-monitoring centers, image compression, data security, and intelligent systems. Teledentistry in the future offers the opportunity to maintain image data banks of whole populations and the possibility of detecting the vast majority of dental disorders very early. In developing countries, where the prevalence of dental disorders is much higher, teledentistry offers the chance to develop very cheap methods of screening for dental disorders with portable digital imaging equipment operated by dental hygienists and ubiquitous health workers throughout the community.

For widespread use, teledentistry systems need to develop economic reality through a reimbursement formula from government health and insurance agencies so that health workers everywhere can take on these responsibilities in addition to their already stretched workloads. A wholesome program of community awareness on the nature and dangers of dental disorders needs to be carried out to induce the whole population to participate in screenings even if they think their conditions are normal. Dentists and dental hygienists need to be convinced that teledentistry will be a powerful addition to their expertise rather than a faceless competitor.

In a very short time, the field of teledentistry has become extensive to be covered by one or two experts. Consequently, this book encapsulates global efforts in the development of teledentistry with contributions from many international experts with first-hand experience. Their contributions in the not-too-distant future will be seen as major developments in dental care. My guiding hope during this task was that as editor of multiple chapters, we could still write with a single voice and keep the content coherent and simple. I hope that the clarity of this book makes up for any limitations in its comprehensiveness.

I would like to thank all authors for making this book possible through their contributions. I took much care that this book would not be merely a collection of separate chapters but rather offer a consistent and structured overview of the field. I am aware that there is still considerable room for improvement and that certain elements of teledentistry are not fully covered, such as legal and reimbursement policy. I invite readers to send comments and feedback to further improve and expand future editions of this book.

Memphis, TN, USA Sajeesh Kumar, PhD

Contents

1 Electronic Health Records in Dentistry: Clinical Challenges and Ethical Issues 1
Robert Cederberg, Muhammad Walji, and John Valenza

2 Teledentistry and the Distant Diagnosis of Oral Mucosal Disease 13
Cassius C. Torres-Pereira, Imara de Almeida Castro Morosini, and Bruna Basso Fonseca

3 Potential Caries Assessment Methods for Teledentistry 23
Robert S. Jones

4 Home Telecare Program on Oral Health 35
Hon K. Yuen

5 Teledentistry-Assisted Affiliated Practice Dental Hygiene 43
Fred F. Summerfelt

6 Teledentisry and Dental Hygiene 53
Tracye A. Moore

7 Access to Oral Care Through Teledentistry 65
Susan J. Daniel and Sajeesh Kumar

8 Forensic Odontology in Digital Era 75
Kelly Tanner Williams and Brenda Tallon Bradshaw

9 Teledentistry in Brazil 87
Mary Caroline Skelton-Macedo, Ana Estela Haddad, and João Humberto Antoniazzi

10 Teleconsultation and Telediagnosis for Oral Health Assessment: An Australian Perspective 101
Rodrigo Mariño, K. Clarke, D.J. Manton, A. Stranieri, R. Collmann, H. Kellet, and A. Borda

Index 113

Contributors

Imara de Almeida Castro Morosini Department of Stomatology, Federal University of Paraná, Curitiba, Paraná, Brazil

João Humberto Antoniazzi Health and Biomedical Informatics Centre, Melbourne Medical School, University of Melbourne, Australia

A. Borda Health and Biomedical Informatics Centre, Melbourne Medical School, University of Melbourne, Australia

Brenda T. Bradshaw Associate Professor Rodrigo MariñoPrincipal Research FellowOral Health Cooperative Research CentreMelbourne Dental School, The University of Melbourne, Melbourne, Australia

Robert Cederberg, DDS Department of General Practice and Dental Public Health, University of Texas School of Dentistry at Houston, Houston, TX, USA

K. Clarke Institute for a Broadband-Enabled Society, University of Melbourne, Melbourne, Australia

R. Collmann Victorian eResearch Strategic Initiative, University of Melbourne, Melbourne, Australia

Susan J. Daniel, RDH, PhD Chairman and Associate Professor, G.W. Hirschfeld School of Dental Hygiene, 2011 College of Health Sciences, Old Dominion University, Norfolk, VA, USA

Bruna Basso Fonseca Department of Stomatology, Federal University of Paraná, Curitiba, Paraná, Brazil

Ana Estela Haddad Department of Paediatrics, Teledentistry Centre, School of Dentistry, University of São Paulo, São Paulo, Brazil

Robert S. Jones Division of Pediatric Dentistry, School of Dentistry, University of Minnesota, Minneapolis, MN, USA

H. Kellet Oral Health Cooperative Research Centre, Melbourne Dental School, The University of Melbourne, Melbourne, Australia

Sajeesh Kumar, PhD Department of Health Informatics and Information Management, University of Tennessee Health Science Center, Memphis, TN, USA

D.J. Manton Oral Health Cooperative Research Centre, Melbourne Dental School, The University of Melbourne, Melbourne, Australia

Rodrigo Mariño Principal, Research Fellow, Oral Health Cooperative Research Centre, Melbourne Dental School, The University of Melbourne, Melbourne, VIC, Australia

Tracye A. Moore, RDH, MS, EdD Dental Hygiene Department, Northern Arizona University, Flagstaff, AZ, USA

Mary Caroline Skelton-Macedo Department of Dentistry-Telehealth/ Teledentistry Centre, Dental School-University of São Paulo, São Paulo, Brazil

A. Stranieri Centre for Informatics and Applied Optimisation, University of Ballarat, Ballarat, Australia

Fred F. Summerfelt, RDH, MEd Department of Dental Hygiene, Northern Arizona University, Flagstaff, AZ, USA

Cassius C. Torres-Pereira, DDS, PhD Department of Stomatology, Federal University of Paraná, Curitiba, Paraná, Brazil

John Valenza Department of General Practice and Dental Public Health, University of Texas School of Dentistry at Houston, Houston, TX, USA

Muhammad Walji Diagnostic and Biomedical Sciences, University of Texas School of Dentistry at Houston, Houston, TX, USA

Kelly Tanner Williams, RDH, MSDH Old Dominion University, Gene W. Hirschfeld School of Dental Hygiene, Norfolk, VA, USA

Hon K. Yuen, PhD, OTR/L Department of Occupational Therapy, School of Health Professions, University of Alabama at Birmingham, Birmingham, AL, USA

Chapter 1
Electronic Health Records in Dentistry: Clinical Challenges and Ethical Issues

Robert Cederberg, Muhammad Walji, and John Valenza

Abstract Today Electronic Health Records (EHRs) have enjoyed wide spread adoption as the optimal choice for the management of patient health information (PHI). EHRs provide several distinct advantages over the use of paper records or a combination of electronic and hard copy options. The ability to interconnect the convenience of computer and software functionality with large amounts of PHI which must be managed for all patients who are being treated by a myriad of health care professionals, including dentists, makes the marriage of electronic data management with the patient record a logical choice. However, the use of EHRs in hospitals, institutions, clinics and private practices also presents many clinical challenges, as well as the potential for a breach in ethical patient care. This chapter discusses the impact of bringing the computer into the patient treatment arena and its effect on the doctor patient relationship, the privacy and security of PHI, ethical issues and clinical challenges, the use of EHRs for research and development of cloud-based EHRs, as well as the future of this technology.

Keywords Electronic Health Records • Doctor-Patient relationship • Privacy • Security • Confidentiality • Ethics • Secondary Use • Data Repository • Cloud-Based EHR

1.1 Introduction

Electronic Health Records (EHRs) have become a common practice management tool for most of today's dental offices and dental clinics. EHRs facilitate the management of large amounts of data and allow the practitioner a means with which to control what used to be a mountain of paper that made up the patient's record.

R. Cederberg, DDS (✉) • J. Valenza
Department of General Practice and Dental Public Health, University of Texas School of Dentistry at Houston, 7500 Cambridge St, Suite 6350, Houston, TX 77054, USA
e-mail: robert.a.cederberg@uth.tmc.edu

M. Walji
Diagnostic and Biomedical Sciences, University of Texas School of Dentistry at Houston, Houston, TX, USA

S. Kumar (ed.), *Teledentistry*, Health Informatics,
DOI 10.1007/978-3-319-08973-7_1

Few would question that EHRs have become a tremendous timesaver and an irreplaceable adjunct to the health care practices of the twenty-first century. However, for all of the benefits that the EHR has provided there are still many challenges and ethical issues that have been created by the use of the EHR in health care. For example, EHRs may increase a clinician's legal responsibility and accountability to be more intimately familiar with the entire content of the record, and as the accessibility and portability of patient data is enhanced ethical dilemmas will likely increases as EHRs become more interconnected and widely used [1].

Healthcare in general has embraced EHR technology for many obvious advantages: (1) less paper to manage, (2) frees up storage space, (3) better tracking and management of patient data, (4) digital imaging, (5) electronic claims, (6) accounting and (7) reporting functionality. The evolution of dental informatics, proliferation of dental information on the internet, increased accessibility of evidenced based dentistry for the practitioner, and accessibility of extensive databases such as MEDLINE have put the computer and EHRs at the forefront of the technology today in the practice of medicine and dentistry today.

Other driving forces in the widespread adoption of the EHRs in dentistry are the changes that are occurring in health care on a national level. The American Recovery and Reinvestment Act (ARRA) put pressure on hospitals to comply with implementation of EHRs or face penalties in Medicaid payments [2]. The Health Information Technology for Economic and Clinical Health (HITECH) Act of 2009 provided further incentives to health care providers to adopt EHRs and in 2011 the Medicare Electronic Health Records Incentive Program for the Centers for Medicare and Medicaid Services began providing incentive payments for the "meaningful" use of EHRs [3]. These laws have had a significant impact on the entire health care system, including office-based physicians and dentists [3]. As of 2012, 72 % of physicians had adopted some form of EHR in their offices [4]. Although there are no current studies for the rate of adoption of the EHR in dental offices, it is likely that it has progressed at a similar rate to physicians.

All of these factors have propelled and accelerated the implementation of EHRs by hospitals, clinics and offices. With this growth comes magnification of the ethical issues, privacy risks and clinical challenges. Sharing patient information through the EHR between providers allows for more flexibility, time savings and instantaneous access to important health information. However, clinicians must practice basic ethical principles such as avoiding harm to others, working diligently to protect patient privacy and developing clinical protocols that will address the challenges that bringing the computer and the EHR into the patient treatment areas has created [5].

1.2 Computers in Patient Treatment Areas

1.2.1 Chairside Use of the EHR in Dentistry

Computers now have a consistent presence within the dental operatory after initially being found only in the front desk area of many dental offices. With the advent of EHRs convenience has driven the movement of the computer to a chair-side location due to the need to enter patient information such as tooth charting, access to a patient's health information including the medical history, development and display of the treatment plan, radiographic capture and display, intraoral photography, prescription writing and patient education to name just a few of the chair-side computing functions that are critical to patient treatment. Schleyer in 2004 reported that about 25 % of the nation's general dentists employed a computer in the dental operatory [6]. As of 2006 the American Dental Association reported that this percentage had more than doubled in a 2 year span [7]. There is no contemporary data to support an estimate of the number of computers utilized in dental operatories today, but it would be safe to assume that chair-side computing has become a mainstream adoption in the modern dental office. However, academic dental schools have rapidly adopted EHRs into their patient care clinics [8–10].

Computers made their first appearance in the dental operatory in the 1980s with the advent of intraoral cameras [11]. These proprietary applications were stand alone and did not offer the benefit of integration with other patient record functions, so they were not well accepted by the dentist. The first truly integrated patient record systems for dentistry arrived in the 1990s and offered a complement to patient record functionality. However; most dental practices maintained hybrid records during this time because many functions, such as radiographs, had not yet been integrated into the EHR. The 2000s brought further evolution of the EHR which allowed for dental offices to become "paperless" for the first time. Today there are a multitude of EHRs on the market all of which offer sophisticated administrative functionality along with all of the clinical features that should be a part of a comprehensive EHR. All of these systems can capture and store images or are well integrated with PACs systems for the management of images. Additionally, some of these systems have broad adaptability that allow usage in a small dental offices up to and including large dental schools, institutions or anything in-between. Today's EHRs used in dentistry are quite robust and manufacturers are continually adjusting these systems to best fit the needs of the dentist and the patient.

Interconnectivity of EHRs between hospitals, physicians, dentists and other health care workers is expected to reduce the inefficiencies with patient care, reduce costs and improve outcomes. Being able to connect with a patient's health record, as well as a patient's complete treatment history from all current and past providers chair-side, should provide the dentist with the best and most up-to-date medical and dental information for their patient. Obviously, this should provide a significant treatment advantage for the dentist, as well as providing the patient a feeling of confidence in their dentist [7]. The American Dental Association is working on a dental component that will be integrated into medical EHRs, so that dentistry will be represented in future EHR development so that all health care disciplines will be represented in a comprehensive health record [7]. With 2015 fast approaching the concept of interconnectivity will likely drive the evolution of EHRs to be inclusive of all aspects of health care, including dentistry.

1.2.2 *Impact of the EHR on the Doctor-Patient Relationship*

It has been suggested the presence of the computer in the dental operatory has introduced a new dynamic to the doctor-patient relationship [12]. The effects of the EHR in the operatory on the doctor-patient relationship has been investigated and it has been found that providers show three distinct types of practice styles when using an EHR as they interact with patients. They position themselves at the computer monitor and concentrate on computer monitor displayed data, or they stand or sit away from the computer and face the patient, or they alternate their attention in defined intervals between the patient and the computer [13]. Especially when the computer is not within the immediate treatment area the provider must divert his/her attention from the patient or as show in Figure 1.1 a second person is needed to enter patient data during an examination (Fig. 1.1). Placement of the computer within the immediate treatment area does allow for better interaction with the patient, but in any of these positions, regardless of the amount of attention paid to the patient, the computer effectively pulls the doctor away from being fully attentive to the patient (Fig. 1.2). Patients want to be involved in their own care and the ability to display patient information on a monitor helps to keep the patient engaged, but there is also a fine line between holding patient interest and alienating the patient through interaction with the computer.

The doctor-patient relationship has always been viewed as a dyad, i.e. the professional (doctor) versus the vulnerable patient with the doctor owing certain duties to the patient [14]. With the advent of EHRs and the desire to create personal health records, patient information has been shared amongst providers and has added another straining point to the doctor-patient relationship. If the use of EHRs becomes ubiquitous and the interconnectivity of a patient's health information becomes widespread, then how much say should patients have with how their information is shared?

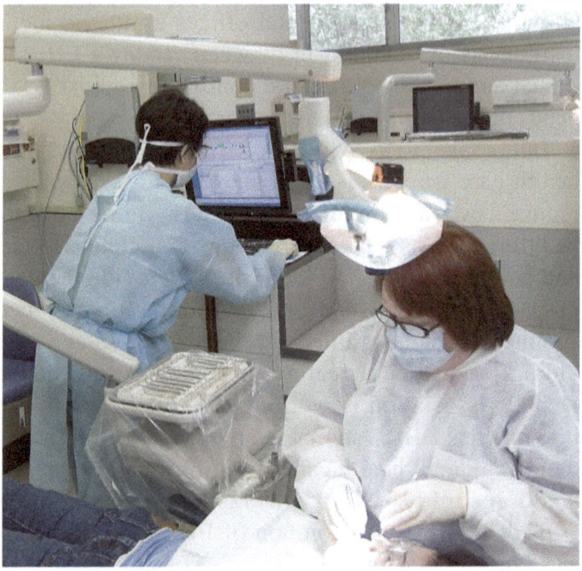

Fig. 1.1 The positioning of the computer and monitor away from the immediate treatment area does not allow for direct interaction with the patient when collecting data during an examination, and as is demonstrated in the photo, may require both an examiner an assistant for data entry

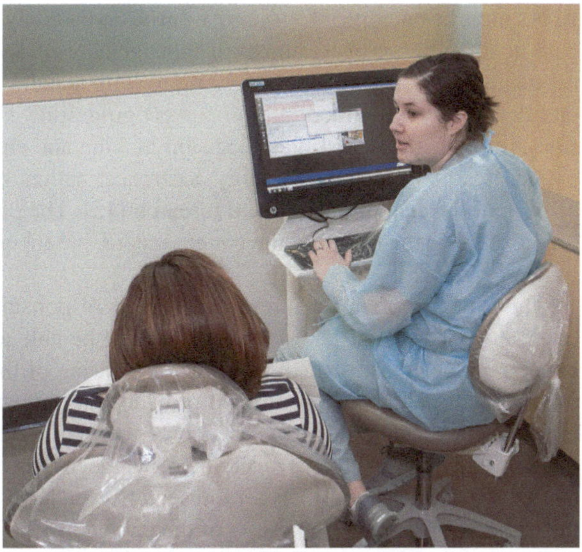

Fig. 1.2 Placement of the monitor and/or all-in-one computer within the patient treatment arena allows the provider to have direct interaction with the patient during patient intake, recording medical history and performing the oral examination

The interconnectivity and the use of patient health information across providers and disciplines is an important public health concern. The ability to create an early-warning system for public health emergencies through use of interconnected EHRs becomes a public health benefit [14]. There needs to be a balance between the good of the patient and the good of the public when it comes to the sharing of patient data.

All health care providers have an obligation to their patients to record, monitor and track data related to patient health. With the advent of the EHR this can be done seamlessly and will allow the provider the ability to track and monitor numerous parameters of health. Additionally, clinicians have the moral duty to report or disclose certain general conditions of health that may affect the public at large [14]. For example, if a particular physician sees an increase in certain variety of influenza he or she would have the duty to report it to a public health agency. As personal health records and EHRs become widely interconnected the clinician and the patient will need to come to an understanding of how patient information is used and shared. For this to be universally accepted the clinician and the patient must allow technology to be used for the public good. There is reason to believe that this will be well accepted by both health care providers and patients and hopefully this technology will strengthen not weaken the doctor-patient relationship.

1.3 Privacy, Security and Confidentiality Issues with EHR Use in Dentistry

The patient record, whether it is a paper copy or an electronic version, is the business record of the health care system. Patients have the right to keep information about themselves from being disclosed to others. Computer systems that house

EHRs must be encrypted for security purposes and only those providers that participate in some phase of treatment or management of the patient should be allowed access to the patient record according to long standing HIPAA (Health Insurance and Portability and Accountability Act) guidelines. The EHR is a communication tool that supports clinical decision making and encompasses many aspects of patient treatment including quality assurance, patient education, and coordination of treatment, legal protection and research [15]. The physician, dentist, practice or organization is the owner of the patient record, but the patient owns the information in the record [15].

The patient or their legal representative is responsible for the care, custody and control of the EHR [16]. Adult patients must be able to make their own decisions concerning healthcare which includes the sharing of their health information with other entities. They must be able to provide consent when their health information is to be shared with an entity outside of the practice that is providing their care. When a patient is unable to make their own decisions concerning their care due to age or some incapacity then a representative or legal guardian must make these decisions within the best interests of the patient [16].

The increased use of EHRs has also increased concerns for the security of patient's health information. Additionally, the widespread use of mobile devices such as smartphones has heightened concerns from information technology consultants that confidential patient information can be compromised. The HITECH Act mandates that the Department of Health and Human Services conduct periodic security audits of health care providers, as well as their business associates [17]. Although the odds of a practice or clinic being audited would be low at least, this threat should compel health care entities to focus on eliminating potential violations which would include data safeguards and other policy and procedural measures to designed to protect the privacy of patient data.

1.4 Ethics and the EHR

When patient health records were strictly paper charts the control of a patient's health information was much easier to manage. With advent of the EHR and the data being entered, stored and retrieved electronically a new level of complexity to controlling this information has been added, as well as presenting conflicts with the ethical principles of beneficence, autonomy, fidelity and justice [18]. Autonomy can be breached when health care data is shared or linked without the patients' knowledge, fidelity can be lost when proper security measures are not applied and justice can be breached when equal access to health information is disparate due to income, literacy, disabilities or other socioeconomic factors [18].

Privacy and confidentiality remain core components of patient rights, but evidence does suggest that the extent of the respect for these rights may be declining [19]. Violations of patient privacy may be easier than ever before because of the efficiency of computerized systems. Thus the potential for a confidentiality breach is increased due to the ease with which data can be replicated and distributed via the computer [19]. Additionally, protecting the privacy of a patient's Protected Health Information (PHI) can be challenging in an electronic environment. These measures often involve the use of unique user IDs and passwords, encryption, remote access controls and computer privacy screens [5]. Protection of PHI involves not only the implementation of measures impacting computer hardware and software, but also on the individual clinician level. Practitioners must be well trained in HIPAA regulations, understand the appropriate ways to manage PHI, understand the issues of shared parenting (consent issues), know what information is appropriate to share with other providers and be aware who is requesting access to PHI [5].

One of the greatest potentials for an ethical breach is in the area of inappropriate access to PHI. Some examples of the issues of access may be: lost or stolen passwords, not properly logging out of computers, not using privacy screens in high patient traffic areas and improper sharing of PHI through e-mail to name just a few. Access of PHI for the purposes of the greater good of the patient has to be balanced against the issue of the personal privacy of the patient [20]. Also, as EHRs and the information contained within the patient record become more widely accessible what groups of providers or ancillary support staff should have access this data and what level of access should be granted? That is, for example, does a laboratory technician, a nurse and a pharmacist, all of whom may participate in a patient's treatment, be provided equal access to the patient's data in the EHR and at what level should this access be? Also, if the patient was diabetic and the pharmacist was prescribing medication would it be helpful for him or her to know the patient's latest HbA1c values? Ultimately, no matter how far technology advances or how interconnected and widespread EHRs become the providers or end-users must still manage the EHR by adhering to sound ethical principles.

1.5 Challenges with the Use of the EHR and Potential Solutions

Along with the proliferation of EHRs have come some challenges that must be met and solutions that must be devised. EHRs provide a way to electronically enter, manage and retrieve large amounts of patient data. Along with the ease of operations in using EHRs comes the ease with which users can create ethical challenges in the way in which patient data is managed. The ease with which previously written clinical or progress notes can be copied and pasted is a potential problem in the record. If there are errors in the text that was copied then those errors will continue to be reproduced [21]. Additionally, if clinic notes are copied from other providers, as may be the case once there is better interconnectivity, then there may not only be errors that may be reproduced, but the issue of plagiarism also becomes a factor.

Another timesaver that is becoming more routinely used is the note template. Practitioners may create a note template that might have standardized language that would be common to a particular oft used procedure. The clinician may often prepopulate the note field with this standardized note and then edit the note following the procedure. Unfortunately, when the clinician is rushed the note may not get properly edited [21]. There are many other shortcuts that can be utilized with EHRs that make record entry and data management much easier for the clinician, but have the potential for pitfalls.

The ability to enter patient data into the EHR chair-side now also makes record entry so much more efficient. As detailed earlier in this chapter, real time data entry, although convenient for the provider, may cause a break in the attention given to the patient. The clinician must constantly divert his or her attention from the patient and onto the computer screen. This break can be perceived by the patient as a lack of attentiveness to their health issues, and secondly the clinician must use his observation skills when asking a patient about his health to see his or her non-verbal reactions. This is an important aspect of medical and dental history taking that may be lost as the doctor-patient relationship is interrupted by the computer [21].

What are some potential solutions? Some clinicians choose to avoid the timesaving aspects that the EHR provides and stick to the meticulous and painstaking methods that we once found as routine when paper records were common place. They avoid using note templates, completely write out patient notes with each visit, refrain from copying and pasting and either write out short notes or type in brief descriptions as the interview patients so they will avoid coming between their patients and the computer [22]. Clinicians ultimately want to practice in a contentious and ethical manner, but also in the most effective and efficient way with the use of the latest technology, so practitioners will need to adapt to the challenges that are introduced by EHRs and computers.

1.6 EHRs and Research

EHRs contain a rich treasure trove of patient data that can be mined for multiple purposes. Clinical researchers may use EHR data to compare treatment outcomes and help establish evidence-based care. Public health researchers may better understand the incidence of dental diseases in specific groups of patients. Dental device companies may find the data useful for helping to determine the frequency of which providers use their products. And payors may use the data to help set reimbursement rates. The use of EHR data for purposes other than for treating and caring for an individual patient is referred to as “secondary use” [23].

While the potential benefits of re-using EHR data are nearly limitless, there are several major challenges [24]. EHR data that are collected as part of the milieu of providing care may not be in a usable format to undergo the rigors of scientific inquiry. Unlike data that are collected as part of clinical trials, EHR data will likely contain differences in both the language and format used by the clinical providers to document patient care. Further, as data are aggregated across different institutions, the variability amongst the sites will be great. For instance a patient’s oral health status may be described in detailed narrative form at one institution, while others

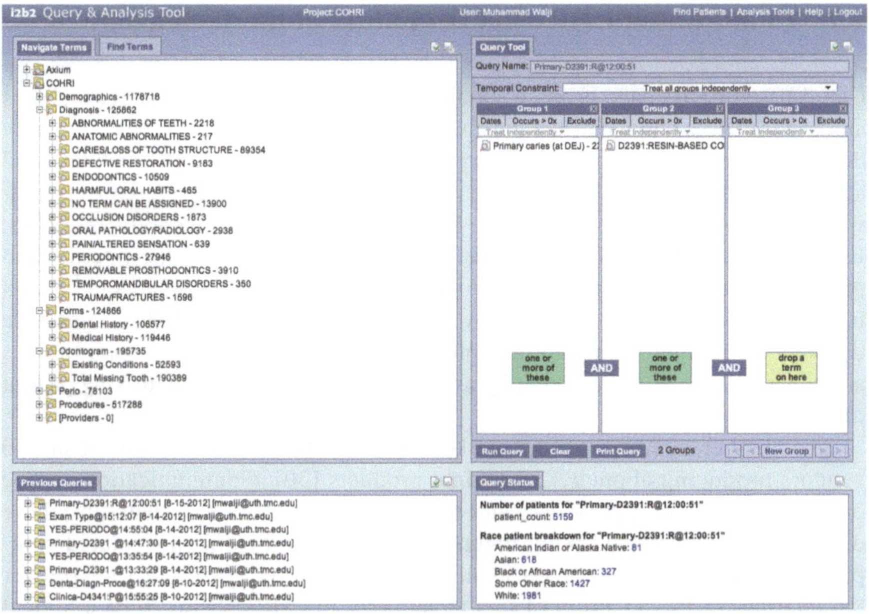

Fig. 1.3 Screen shot of using the Query & Analysis Tool of the BigMouth Dental Data Repository. This tool is based on the i2b2 Data Warehousing platform (i2b2.org) and allows researchers to query de-identified patient data across contributing organizations

may use a neatly placed structured field on a form. To help solve some of these challenges, the Consortium of Oral Health Research and Informatics (COHRI) was founded to provide standardization for how large dental institutions such as dental schools document in an EHR [25]. As a result, many COHRI member institutions now use a consistent medical and dental history form, as well as a standardized dental diagnostic terminology [26]. In addition, a large dental data repository called BigMouth (https://cohri.uth.tmc.edu) has been developed based on data from members of the consortium. Figure 1.3 shows a screen shot from the COHRI project that demonstrates the research power of an EHR database search (Fig. 1.3). This type of search allows the researcher to collect information contained within member institutions EHR databases and provides information on use of treatment codes along with a breakdown of patient demographics.

There are also ethical issues that should also be pondered before reusing patient data for purposes other than direct patient care. First and foremost, patients are often not aware that their data will be reused for secondary purposes [23]. There are some protections in place as part of the Health Insurance Portability and Accountability Act (HIPAA) and specifically the "privacy rule" that sets guidelines for how identifiable patient health information may be used for research purposes and when patient consent is required. However, concerns remain that even when researchers use a fully de-identified dataset there is still a risk of re-identification of patients [27].

1.7 Cloud-Based EHRs and the Future of the Technology

Cloud-based EHRs have become a viable option for health care practices, clinics and even schools and have become an effective method to manage PHI. Not only do cloud-based systems provide a very efficient method to share PHI between and among practitioners, but is also much more cost effective because it reduces hardware costs and licensing fees that are common with client-server software EHRs. Encryption of patient data facilitates information sharing over the internet and provides a means to view PHI in a timely manner which helps patients to be seen in multiple locations on an emergency basis [28]. Cloud-based EHR systems have the potential to improve health care, provide wide reaching research opportunities and to simplify patient treatment by avoiding the duplication of gathering patient data [29].

The number of EHRs on the market continues to grow with more than 700 vendors producing about 1,750 distinct products [30]. Communication among providers or between providers and patients is currently exacerbated by these disparate systems not working together. Current non-health care related companies manage secure and confidential communications with customers over the internet, so the adaption of this technology to EHRs seems to be a logical next step. EHR companies will likely provide bundled, interoperable and suitably adapted technologies that will be optimized for use in the health care environment [30].

1.8 Summary

Many physicians and dentists today continue to be locked into utilization of outmoded EHRs that in some cases were developed years before explosion of the internet. In today's world the need for better, faster and more secure communication is becoming a mandatory aspect of efficient patient treatment. There continues to be a growing need for all providers of health care to be able to effectively communicate with one another and with their patients so that PHI can be securely shared. As information technology and EHRs evolve to allow for more effective patient information management, EHR developers with the help of health care providers need to work together to ensure that these systems, protocols and workflows follow sound principles of data collection, management and storage. EHRs need to be dynamic, state-of-the art and flexible information management systems that allow for patient data to be easily and securely shared and stored, provide sufficient integration of all available clinical applications and be operated in an environment that allows the health care practitioner to deliver care that is evidence-based and provided in a manner that is ethically sound.

References

1. Sittig DF, Singh H. Legal ethical, and financial dilemmas in electronic health record adoption and use. Pediatrics. 2011;127(4):e1042–7.
2. Bigalke JT. Filling the healthcare IT gap by 2015. Healthc Financ Manage. 2009;63(6):38–40.
3. Kalenderian E, Walji M, Ramoni R. "Meaningful use" of EHR in dental school clinics: how to benefit from the U.S. HITECH act's financial and quality improvement incentives. J Dent Educ. 2013;77(4):401–15.
4. Hsiaa C, Jha AK, King J, Patel V, Furukawa MF, Mostashari F. Office-based physicians are responding to incentives and assistance by adopting and using electronic health records. Health Aff. 2013;32(8):1470–7.
5. Neilsen BA, Baum RA, Soares NS. Navigating ethical issues with electronic health records I developmental-behavioral pediatric practice. J Dev Behav Pediatr. 2013;34:45–51.
6. Schleyer T. Why integration is key of dental office technology. J Am Dent Assoc. 2004;135 Suppl 1:4S–9.
7. American Dental Association. 2006 technology survey. Chicago: American Dental Association; 2007.
8. Atkinson JC, Zeller GG, Chhaya S. Electronic patient records for dental school clinics: more than paperless systems. J Dent Educ. 2002;66(5):634–42.
9. Walji MF, Taylor D, Langabeer II JR. Factors influencing implementation and outcomes of a dental electronic patient record system. J Dent Educ. 2009;73(5):589–600.
10. Langabeer II JR, Walji MF, Taylor D, Valenza JA. Economic outcomes of a dental electronic patient record. J Dent Educ. 2008;72(10):1189–200.
11. Sam FE, Bonnick AM. Office computer systems for the dental office. Dent Clin N Am. 2011;55:549–57.
12. Cederberg RA, Valenza JA. Ethics and the electronic health record in dental school clinics. J Dent Educ. 2012;76:584–9.
13. Ventres W, Kooienga S, Vuckovic N, Marlin R, Nygren P, Stewart V. Physicians, patients and the electronic health record: an ethnographic analysis. Ann Fam Med. 2006;4:124–31.
14. Goodman KW. Ethics information technology, and public health: new challenges for the clinician-patient relationship. J Law Med Ethics. 2010;38(1):58–63.
15. Harman LB, Flite CA, Bond K. Electronic health records: privacy, confidentiality, and security. Virtual Mentor. 2012;14(9):712–9. http://virtualmonitor.ama-assn.org//2012/09/stas1-1209.html. Accessed 17 Oct 2013.
16. Kopala B, Mitchell ME. Use of digital health records raises ethics concerns. JONAS Healthc Law Ethics Regul. 2011;13(3):84–9.
17. Greene AH. HHS steps up HIPAA audits: now is the time to review security policies and procedures. J Am Health Inf Manage Assoc. 2011;82(10):58–9.
18. Layman EJ. Ethical issues and the electronic health record. Health Care Manag. 2008;27(2):165–76.
19. Fairweather NB, Rogerson S. A moral approach to electronic patient records. Med Inform. 2001;26(3):219–34.
20. Mick ML, Conners SE. Ethical issue of medical records on the internet. 2010. http://webpages.cs.luc.edu/~laufer/ethics97/papers/MickConners.html. Accessed 16 Dec 2010.
21. Bernat JL. Ethical and quality pitfalls in electronic health records. Neurology. 2013;80(11):1157–61.
22. Avitur A. The worst features of EHRs and how to fix them. Neurol Today. 2012;12169:285–9.
23. Safran C, Bloomrosen M, Hammond WE, Labkoff S, Markel-Fox S, Tang PC, et al. Toward a national framework for the secondary use of health data: an American Medical Informatics Association white paper. J Am Med Inform Assoc. 2007;14(1):1–9.
24. Hersh WR, Weiner MG, Embi PJ, Logan JR, Payne PR, Bernstam EV, et al. Caveats for the use of operational electronic health record data in comparative effectiveness research. Med Care. 2013;51(8 Suppl 3):S30–7.

25. Stark PC, Kalenderian E, White JM, Walji MF, Stewart DC, Kimmes N, et al. Consortium for oral health-related informatics: improving dental research, education, and treatment. J Dent Educ. 2010;74(10):1051–65.
26. Kalenderian E, Ramoni RL, White JM, Schoonheim-Klein ME, Stark PC, Kimmes NS, et al. The development of a dental diagnostic terminology. J Dent Educ. 2011;75(1):68–76.
27. McGraw D. Building public trust in uses of Health Insurance Portability and Accountability Act de-identified data. J Am Med Inform Assoc. 2013;20(1):29–34.
28. Chen Y, Lu J, Jan J. A secure EHR system based on hybrid clouds. 2012. http://link.springer.com/article/10.1007/s10916-012-9830-6/fulltext.html. Accessed 14 Feb 2014.
29. Kuo AM. Opportunities and challenges of cloud computing to improve health care services. J Med Internet Res. 2011;13(3):e67. http://www.ncbi.nlm.nih.gov/pmc/articles/PMC3222190/. Accessed 14 Feb 2014.
30. Mandl KD, Kohane IS. Escaping the EHR trap – the future of health IT. N Engl J Med. 2012. doi:10.1056/NEJMp1203102.

Chapter 2
Teledentistry and the Distant Diagnosis of Oral Mucosal Disease

Cassius C. Torres-Pereira, Imara de Almeida Castro Morosini, and Bruna Basso Fonseca

Abstract Teledentistry can be described as the transmission of synchronous or asynchronous clinical information using electronic health records, digital imaging and telecommunication technology. It can reduce inappropriate referral rates by providing treatment supervision and a second professional opinion based on the exchange of health information. The objective of this chapter is to summarize the telehealth literature in oral medicine and to explore the methods that have been used in this specialty.

Keywords Oral medicine • Oral manifestations • Teledentistry • Telehealth • Medical records

2.1 Introduction

Teledentistry can be considered as the transmission of synchronous or asynchronous clinical information using electronic health records, digital imaging, telecommunication technology and Internet protocols to provide teleconsultations or second opinion with specialists. It can be adopted to guide general practitioners in the distant diagnosis and treatment of common or rare diseases and to reduce inappropriate referral rates by providing treatment supervision and a second professional opinion based on the exchange of health information [1–4].

Some dentistry specialties are experiencing the benefits of the continuing development of telehealth. The practice of teledentistry is expected to reduce economic and emotional costs involved in patient transportation to reference centers, mainly in situations that could be diagnosed or treated in primary-care units. Although the use of telehealth has been studied in many medical specialties, there is a lack of consistent evidence for its advantages in dentistry [1–4].

C.C. Torres-Pereira, DDS, PhD (✉) • I.A.C. Morosini • B.B. Fonseca
Department of Stomatology, Federal University of Paraná,
Curitiba, Paraná, Brazil
e-mail: cassius@ufpr.br

S. Kumar (ed.), *Teledentistry*, Health Informatics,
DOI 10.1007/978-3-319-08973-7_2

Oral medicine is a dentistry specialty devoted to the diagnosis and treatment of oral diseases [5, 6]. Most part of the clinical practice in oral medicine comprises the direct visualization of oral tissues for the recognition of mucosal visible alterations. Visual inspection of the oral mucosa is frequently the first step for the diagnosis and clinical reasoning. It is also the visual inspection that guides the clinician to request complimentary exams or to decide immediately for specific therapeutics. In many parts of the world there is a limited number of oral medicine specialists. It is not rare for patients to delay clinical specialized attention or to have an urgent consultation with professionals outside the oral medicine area [5–7].

In oral medicine, the idea of using teledentistry to triage referrals, and its potential as a tool to support locally based treatment, poses an alternative approach to the management of oral medicine referrals. It has been considered a potentially cost-effective method to provide healthcare to underserved populations, including socially disadvantaged people, those who live in remote or rural areas, where distance from the regional center can be a significant barrier [8–13].

The objective of this chapter is to summarize the telehealth literature in oral medicine and to explore the methods that have been used in this emerging field.

2.2 Telehealth in Oral Medicine: What Is the Evidence?

Many health disciplines, including dentistry, can employ telehealth technologies in the delivery of clinical diagnostic services to remote areas devoid of dental specialists or even general dental practitioners (GDP). Despite this, teledentistry had been rarely used as a method of diagnosis, consultation and referral in dentistry practices [1, 2].

Some studies in dentistry investigated whether the use of internet based communication technology and intraoral cameras for visual oral health screenings would be comparable to traditional screenings [14–16], others developed systems of telemedicine consultation for preoperative assessment or treatments follow up [17–20] and also evaluated patients and clinicians acceptability to these methodologies [8].

Evidence summarized elsewhere shows an increasing number of studies, in different dentistry specialties, which report the use of information technology to improve oral health care [1–4]. Among those studies it is possible to identify reports that investigate the possible practice of oral medicine using a telehealth approach. The concept of oral medicine used in this chapter excludes studies of teledentistry in other fields such as oral radiology, oral maxillofacial surgery and temporomandibular joint disorders and focus in specific research of oral mucosa diseases.

2.2.1 Methods Used for Teleconsultations

Teleconsultations can be conducted basically in two ways: the "store and forward" method or videoconferences. In the "store and forward" method, data collected from oral clinical examinations, oral digital photography or digital radiographic images can be stored in an electronic file format, and all of the patient records can be retrieved and reviewed by specialists using a common electronic platform (Figs. 2.1, 2.2 and 2.3). Alternatively, the data can be sent electronically to another specialist to obtain a second opinion at any time.

In contrast, videoconferences or real time consultations employ direct, on-line computer or satellite telecommunication technologies among specialists and GDP's, telehealth assistants or patients located in remote communities, as long as the specialist remains online to provide instant support and supervision.

Studies have been developed using one or both of these methods depending on the research design and the study objectives but most of them were developed using "store and forward" methodologies. This is probably because they are less expensive and time consuming than videoconferences. A total of six studies in oral medicine are briefly reviewed. They are summarized in Table 2.1.

In the study reported by Leão and Porter [8], the sample was comprised of 20 patients referred to a dental institute for the diagnosis and management of oral mucosal disease. Digital images of oral lesion were captured by intraoral cameras and stored on videotapes, and thus, patients could view their own images on a color monitor. Photographs of each lesion were recorded, printed and stored in the patient's clinical chart. Digital images and important clinical details were recorded in a standardized electronic letter and sent via e-mail as attached files. A group of judges was asked to compare the original and transmitted clinical images and to provide a professional diagnosis of each patient's problem, which was compared to that of the attending consultant. Patients were asked to complete a questionnaire detailing their opinions of intra-oral camera utilization. They also were asked about the acceptability of viewing the images of their lesions.

They concluded that patient and clinician had good acceptability toward recording and electronically transmitting clinical images of common oral diseases and, therefore, aimed to develop the application of this methodology in the distant diagnosis of oral diseases.

Younai and Messadi [9] retrieved 78 complete charts from an oral medicine clinic and blindly evaluated the diagnostic agreement between the final diagnosis (gold standard) and a provisional diagnosis made independently and blinded by two oral medicine specialists based on an email with detailed information from the patients clinical chart. The final diagnosis or clinical hypotheses were omitted from the email. The objective was to test the accuracy of a clinical hypothesis based on the electronic communication of signs and symptoms and other relevant clinical data. The authors were concerned about the legal, ethical and financial impact of the increasing use of electronic communication between the health staff and patients. The authors compare their kappa index to some studies in teledermatology and

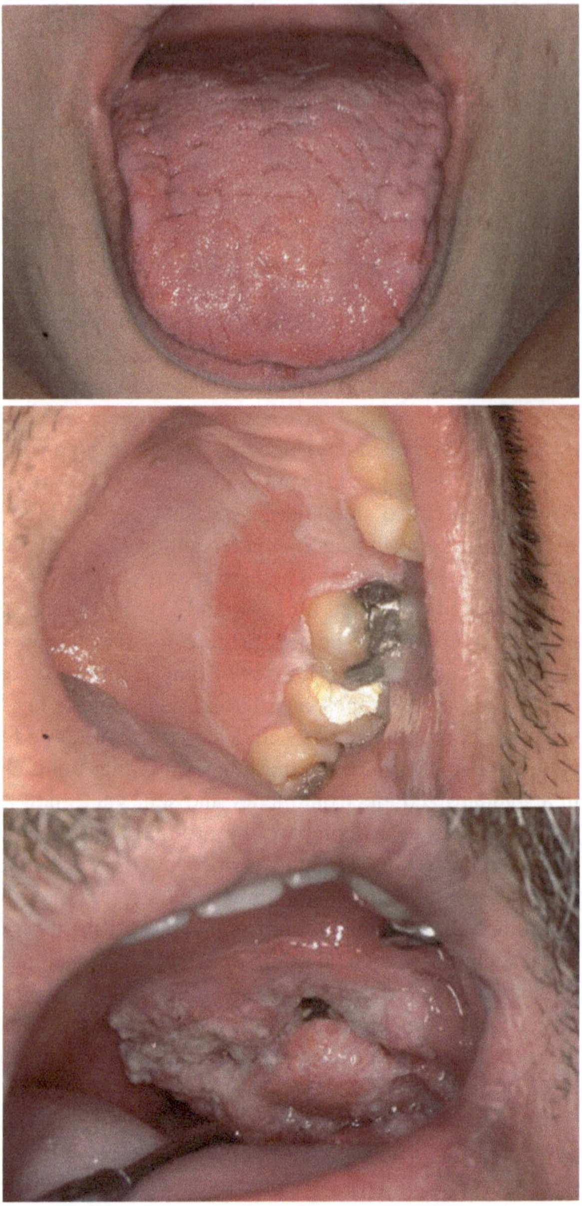

Figs. 2.1, 2.2 and 2.3 Clinical images obtained by a professional camera with macro lens and ring flash: the gold standard for intraoral pictures can have a positive impact in oral medicine cases referral (1. fissured tongue, 2. oral trauma, food burning, 3 oral cancer)

found that even not using clinical pictures of oral lesions there was a moderate level of diagnostic accuracy. Although the impressive kappa results the authors alerted that their pilot study results "suggest that face-to-face patient examination is more accurate in establishing a correct diagnosis for oral mucosal pathologies than transmitted descriptive patient data alone".

Table 2.1 Studies of teledentistry in oral medicine

Reference	Method	N	Conclusion
Leão and Porter [8]	Intraoral camera. Images and resumed clinical history sent by email	20	Patient and clinician showed good acceptability to transmitting clinical images. Appropriate provisional diagnosis in 64 % of cases
Younai and Messadi [9]	Clinical history sent by email. No images of the lesions	71	58–64 % diagnostic agreement between judges and the gold standard
Torres-Pereira et al. [10]	Professional digital camera with macro lens and ring flash. Images and brief clincal history sent by email	25	In 88 % of cases, at least one out of two distant consultants provided the correct diagnosis. Only one case referred for presential specialized consultation.
Bradley et al. [11]	Intraoral camera. Images, and brief clinical history sent by email	37	65 % had clinical common lesions manageable at the primary care facility and 20 % needed urgent hospital visit
Blomstrand et al. [12]	Electronic health records and image Internet-based discussions: "telemedicine rounds".	10	Most patients (n = 8) had the diagnosis and treatment suggested with telemedicine rounds, while two were referred to a specialist.
Torres-Pereira et al. [13]	Professional digital camera with macro lens and ring flash. Images and brief clinical history sent by email	60	In 80 % of cases, at least one out of two distant consultants provided the correct diagnosis

Torres-Pereira et al. [10] studied 25 patients during a 12-month period. All individuals lived in an underserved rural community distant from the main oral medicine reference clinic in southern Brazil. Authors developed an electronic form to record clinical data that was stored as a text-processing file. Oral lesions were documented using a professional digital camera with macro lens and ring flash. The clinical images were saved as JPEG files and then sent as an e-mail attachment to two consultants. Both consultants were oral medicine specialists and evaluated the images blinded and separately. It was requested that they record a maximum of two clinical hypotheses for each case, selected from a predefined list. Final diagnoses (gold standard) were compared to those provided by the remote clinicians to assess the percentage of total, partial or incorrect hypotheses.. The results suggest that digital photography can be an effective alternative in the clinical diagnosis of oral lesions, and primary care public health clinics may benefit from the use of telehealth in remote areas where oral medicine specialists are not available. The authors concluded that there was an acceptable diagnostic accuracy rate with use of oral lesions pictures sent by e-mail and in only one case it was necessary to refer the patient to a major center. They emphasized that the diagnosis of oral lesions using asynchronous technology could be an effective resource to manage referrals in the Brazilian public health system.

Bradley et al. [11] used a prototype teledentistry system as part of a strategy to implement a teledentistry service in Northern Ireland. The prototype included a personal computer and an intraoral camera. The study was conducted in Belfast with 37 patients. The feasibility of distance-diagnosis of oral mucosal diseases through e-mail and a store-and-forward image system was investigated using transmission of digital images to distant consultants. The authors identified that 8 (20 %) out of the 37 referred patients should be seen in person and the others (65 %) could be treated or monitored at the primary care facility under supervision of the remote oral medicine expert. The teledentistry system identified also one "harmless lesion" and one case of referral to the wrong specialty. The authors described that the system was "especially suitable for management of referrals of older dependant adults who have oral mucosal disease". They found that teledentistry may represent a cost effective approach to manage referrals in oral medicine.

Blomstrand et al. [12] investigated an interactive system for Internet-based consultations and discussions via "telemedicine rounds", which was tested in a pilot study with 10 patients. The system consisted of a secure Internet-based application, standard personal computers, broadband Internet connections, and a digital camera. They used vocal communication by conference phones. As a result, 8 patients had the diagnosis and treatment suggested in the telemedicine rounds, while only 2 were referred to a specialist. The dental health clinic could thus provide treatment without the need for referral to a consultant. They concluded that telemedicine system described allows patient care to be provided rapidly and more economically.

Torres-Pereira et al. (2013) repeated their accuracy study using the digital professional camera with macro lens and ring flash for oral mucosa pictures. They increased the sample to 60 patients that had their lesions images and their most important clinical informations attached to emails sent to two distant consultants. The results were similar to the their first pilot study where the two consultants made up to 80 % correct clinical hypotheses when compared to the final histopathology description (gold standard).

The use of Internet in telehealth may be a practical mean of communication between dental clinicians, thereby improving patient management. Considering the evidence available, teledentistry consultation in oral medicine can be considered quite as reliable as traditional visits. It has the advantage of being an efficient and probably more economical method for providing preoperative assessments when patient transportation is difficult or costly. It is plausible that teledentistry also can improve access to diagnosis and treatment for those who would otherwise not receive an immediate and early care.

Information technology could increase the accuracy of consultations because it allows the specialist to review digital images outside of a medical center quickly and easily and could provide a screening method to organize a referral system for patients requiring specialty services. It can improve the efficiency of specialty triaging and allows the integration of remote experts, thus facilitating the global availability of specialized knowledge (Figs. 2.4, 2.5 and 2.6).

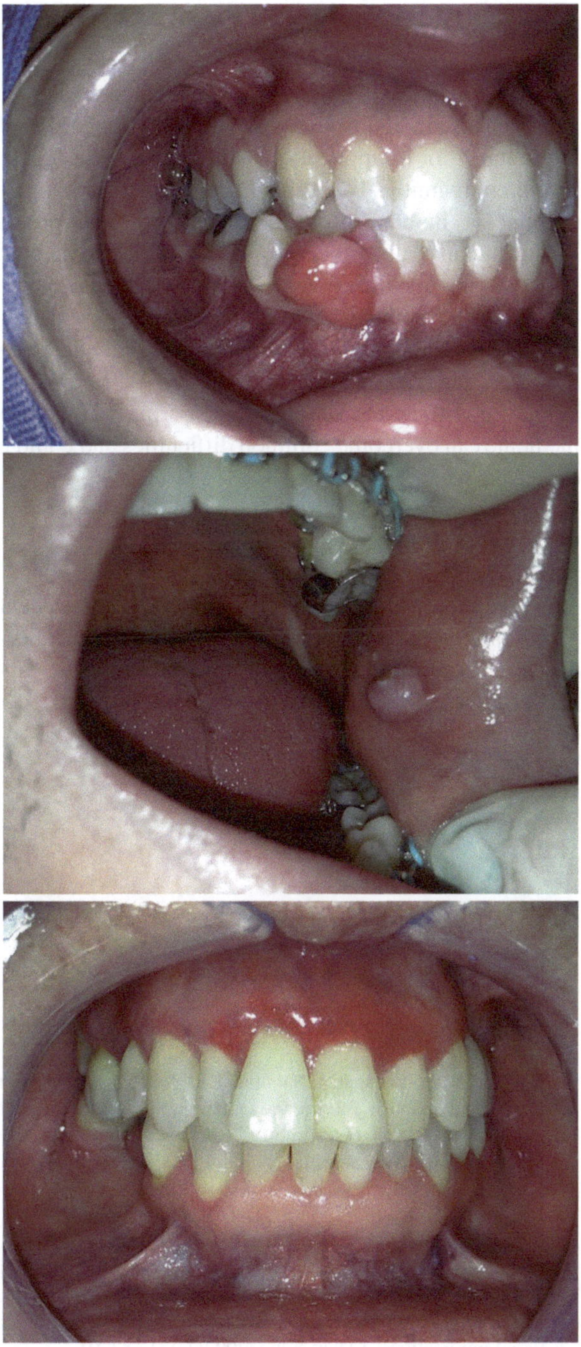

Figs. 2.4, 2.5 and 2.6 Clinical images obtained by a smartphone camera can provide good clinical pictures for the preliminar appraisal and the chart register of clinical oral manifestations. (1. peripheral ossifying fibroma, 2. fibroma, 3. mucous membrane pemphigoid)

2.3 Considerations and Future Directions

This brief review has demonstrated that teledentistry is being considered a feasible approach also in oral medicine; however, a standard method or minimum equipment requirement for its application in the specialty has not yet been established. Distinct health communities can experience distinct problems such as the availability and training of human resources, bandwidth and protocols of data transmission. Financial constraints in developing countries should be a concern. Also, it is worth remembering that the implementation of a teledentistry system can be more difficult outside the academia where time and training are usually less problematic than in a non academic outpatient public or private practice. Nevertheless, in some studies, low cost and domestic technologies such as digital cameras and e-mail were employed with good results, demonstrating that the benefits of teledentistry in oral medicine can overcome common difficulties and could be experienced even without expensive resources.

Some medical specialties are developing faster in telehealth research. In dentistry it can be observed an increasing research output in areas such as oral and maxillofacial surgery, orthodontics, pediatric dentistry and special care dentistry. Oral medicine seems to be a promising area for teledentistry investigation.

Despite the impressive evolution of communication technology in the last two decades, it seems reasonable to direct future investigations toward determining the barriers that still delay the implementation of teledentistry as an adjunct for a comprehensive health care system.

References

1. Daniel SJ, Wu L, Kumar S. Teledentistry: a systematic review of clinical outcomes, utilization and costs. J Dent Hyg. 2013;87(6):345–52.
2. Mariño R, Ghanim A. Teledentistry: a systematic review of the literature. J Telemed Telecare. 2013;19:179–83.
3. Khan SA, Omar H. Teledentistry in practice: literature review. Telemed J E Health. 2013;19:565–7.
4. Jampani ND, Nutalapati R, Dontula BS, Boyapati R. Applications of teledentistry: a literature review and update. J Int Soc Prev Community Dent. 2011;1(2):37–44. Review.
5. Sollecito TP, Rogers H, Prescott-Clements L, Felix DH, Kerr AR, Wray D, Shirlaw P, Brennan MT, Greenberg MS, Stoopler ET. Oral medicine: defining an emerging specialty in the United States. J Dent Educ. 2013;77(4):392–4. Review.
6. Rogers H, Sollecito TP, Felix DH, Yepes JF, Williams M, D'Ambrosio JA, Hodgson TA, Prescott-Clements L, Wray D, Kerr AR. An international survey in postgraduate training in oral medicine. Oral Dis. 2011;17 Suppl 1:95–8. doi:10.1111/j.1601-0825.2011.01785.x.
7. Sardella A, Demarosi F, Lodi G, Canegallo L, Rimondini L, Carrassi A. Accuracy of referrals to a specialist oral medicine unit by general medical and dental practitioners and the educational implications. J Dent Educ. 2007;71(4):487–91.
8. Leão J, Porter S. Telediagnosis of oral disease. Braz Dent J. 1999;10(1):47–53.

9. Younai FS, Messadi DV. E-mail-based oral medicine consultation. J Calif Dental Assoc. 2000;28:144–51.
10. Torres-Pereira C, Possebon RS, Simões A, Bortoluzzi MC, Leão JC, Giovanini AF, Piazetta CM. Email for distance diagnosis of oral diseases: a preliminar study of teledentistry. J Telemed Telecare. 2008;14:435–8.
11. Bradley M, Black P, Noble S, Thompson R, Lamey PJ. Application of teledentistry in oral medicine in a community dental service. N Ireland Br Dent J. 2010;209:399–404.
12. Blomstrand L, Gullbrandsson L, Kildal M. Telemedicine – a complement to traditional referrals in oral medicine. Telemed J E Health. 2012;18:549–53.
13. Torres-Pereira C, Morosini IAC, Possebon RS, Bortoluzzi MC, Leão JC, Piazzeta CM. Teledentistry: distant diagnosis of oral disease using e-mails. Telemed J E Health. 2013;19:117–21.
14. Patterson S, Botchway C. Dental screenings using telehealth technology: a Pilot Study. J Can Dent Assoc. 1998;64:806–10.
15. Kopycka-Kedzierawski DT, Billings RJ, McConnochie KM. Dental screening of preschool children using teledentistry: a feasibility study. Pediatr Dent. 2007;29(3):209–13.
16. Kopycka-Kedzierawski DT, Billings RJ. Teledentistry in inner-city child-care centres. J Telemed Telecare. 2006;12(4):176–81.
17. Rollert MK, Strauss RA, Abubaker AO, Hampton C. Telemedicine consultations in oral and maxillofacial surgery. J Oral Maxillofac Surg. 1999;57:136–8.
18. Nickenig H, Wichmann M, Schlegel A, Eitner S. Use of telemedicine for pre-implant dental assessment – a comparative study. J Telemed Telecare. 2008;14(2):93–7.
19. Ewers R, Schicho K, Wagner A, et al. Seven years of clinical experience with teleconsultation in craniomaxillofacial surgery. J Oral Maxillofac Surg. 2005;63:1447–54.
20. Aziz SR, Ziccardi VB. Telemedicine using smartphonesfor oral and maxillofacial surgery consultation, communication and treatment planning. J Oral Maxillofac Surg. 2009;67:2505–9.

Chapter 3
Potential Caries Assessment Methods for Teledentistry

Robert S. Jones

Abstract This chapter focuses on caries detection and optical based imaging technologies that have the potential to be used for oral health screening of children and adults by adjunct personnel. Another focus is examining how teledentistry based caries detection needs to be integrated with risk assessment and topical management approaches. This chapter also focuses on the importance of using a teledentistry lesion scale (TLS) where assessment scores directly correlate to clinical recommendations in order to simply the work flow in teledentistry. This chapter discusses the evidence of scattering and fluorescence based optical caries detection systems in the context of teledentistry. Despite considerable advancements in the technology of early caries detection, advanced imaging and detection methods have not been shown to have markedly superior diagnostic values from simple visual image analysis for use in teledentistry.

Keywords Caries Management • Teledentistry Lesion Scale • Optical Scattering Detection Systems • Cross-Polarization Optical Coherence Tomography • Fluorescence-based Optical Detection Systems

Optimal oral health care benefits from the detection of early changes in health. For this chapter, dental caries, especially in children will be the primary focus. For dental caries, the most optimal oral health care is identifying caries risk factors and the presence or absence of protective factors and practices [1]. This assessment can be integrated with a teledentistry based oral health screening delivered by adjunct dental personal, who can deliver preventive dental care. With the new adoption of mid-level providers (e.g. dental therapists), teledentistry can also assist with restorative care in children and less advanced restorative care in adults. Diagnostic imaging methods have the potential to be used by mid-level providers to offsite dentists for real-time perioperative evaluation and post-procedure quality assurance programs.

R.S. Jones
Division of Pediatric Dentistry, School of Dentistry, University of Minnesota,
6-150 Moos Health Science Tower, 515 Delaware Street S.E., Minneapolis, MN 55455, USA
e-mail: rsjones@umn.edu

S. Kumar (ed.), *Teledentistry*, Health Informatics,
DOI 10.1007/978-3-319-08973-7_3

3.1 Caries Management

Strategies for managing dental caries have increasingly used the concept of risk assessment [2, 3]. Caries risk assessment is the determination of the likelihood incidence of caries in the immediate future. Importantly, preventive dental care has the potential to be delivered by adjunct dental personnel in remote or critical access areas. Children with a high-risk for dental caries may be effectively screened for early presence of non-cavitated lesions utilizing telehealth technologies [4]. Children can be screened with an intraoral camera in teledentistry where images are collected by trained adjunct dental personnel. Images can then be interpreted and assessed by an offsite dentist. Teledentistry may also include caries risk assessment questionnaires and objective caries detection measurements that are forwarded to a dentist for a comprehensive evaluation. Although most questionnaires based risk assessment do not have high diagnostic predictively, without using bacteria screening [5–7], risk assessment is a critical step in teledentistry. For example, children who are exposed to community water fluoridation are not only less likely to have dental decay but their overall severity is less [8]. Risk assessment also reinforces the teledentistry focus on evaluating the overall oral health of the patient and not solely examining individual teeth.

Caries risk also aims to predict the rate of progression of current non-cavitated carious lesions [9]. The dental team can help prevent cavitation of early incipient enamel lesions by correctly identifying key risk factors and demineralization in the early stages [10, 11]. The presence of non-cavitated lesions have been shown to have a predictive value for future caries elsewhere [12]. Detecting near-surface incipient lesions allow arresting or reversing the disease progression through topical therapies and improved oral hygiene and diet, as highlighted in CAMBRA caries management strategies [12, 13]. For patients with incipient non-cavitated lesions that have progressed just into the outer surface of dentin, sealant placement or minimal invasive restorations are advantageous to arrest the lesion [14]. Risk assessment is now viewed as the critically important step in the clinical decision process of managing the disease. For teledentistry, caries risk assessment can effectively manage and triage patients for treatment planning, prevention, and establishing follow-up and recall times.

3.2 Teledentistry Lesion Scale (TLS)

Several authors have recognized the importance of integrating caries detection and assessment with clinical treatment recommendations [15, 16]. Most assessment methods attempt to measure dental caries along the continuum of the disease. Common oral radiology assessment evaluates and scores lesion progression by

Table 3.1 Teledentistry Lesion Scale (TLS)

Score	0	1	2
Gold standard assessment	Sound, no evidence of demineralization	Demineralization extending into enamel only	Demineralization extending into enamel and outer dentin
CAMBRA based recommendations	Assess/address	Assess/address risk factors	Assess/address risk factors
	Risk factors	Arrest/remin early lesion with therapeutics	Treat with minimal intervention (e.g. sealant or small restoration)

progression in depth. For example, dentist will score and record enamel lesions confined either to the outer half (E1) versus approaching the enamel-dentin junction (E2). Visual assessment (ICDAS-II) of occlusal surfaces attempts to capture the different stages of the disease progression [17–19]. Newer adjunct detection systems have modeled their assessment from these radiographic and visual assessment ordinal scales of diagnostic criteria [16, 20]. The benefits of a larger dynamic range of scoring allow dentists to measure disease progression and rate; however, there is still little longitudinal trials evaluating the ability to monitor carious lesion progression using these scoring systems. In terms of teledentistry, compressing any scoring system benefits the logistics and workflow of providing oral care. The teledentistry lesion scale (TLS) is a simple scoring method where tooth structure is scored 0–2. Its purpose is to simplify the treatment triage decision making process in teledentistry. TLS uses a scoring method that is related directly with possible clinical recommended treatment options (Table 3.1). This methodology is similar to those employed by past studies examining how lesion assessment translates to treatment decisions by an examiner [21, 22]. A score 0 indicates that the tooth appears sound with no evidence of demineralization. This corresponds to a CAMBRA recommendation to address the presence or absence of risk factors and protective factors [13, 23, 24]. A score '1' indicates that an examiner identifies the presence of an enamel-only caries lesion. The likely treatment option applied clinically would be to determine key biological and behavior risk factors and consider topical therapies (e.g. fluoride based) to promote lesion remineralization [13, 23, 24]. This preventive treatment can be delivered by adjunct dental personnel remotely. A score '2' indicates that demineralization has progressed into the dentin. The likely treatment option would be to determine risk factors for future caries, deliver appropriate prevention therapy, and seal or restore the lesion with the most minimal intervention possible [23, 25]. In certain circumstances, a midlevel provider can provide care to children or an adult in a critical access area. This would be done after final assessment and treatment planning by a dentist.

3.3 Caries Detection Methods

Caries on fissured surfaces account for over 80 % of all caries on young permanent teeth [26]. Dental radiography may not effectively identify early non-cavitated lesions on critical tooth surfaces. Occlusal caries continue to be difficult to identify and monitor, particularly in the early stages, using conventional methodologies. The nature of dental decay, especially pits and fissure caries, has changed dramatically with the use of fluoride, where lesions are often *hidden* underneath an intact veneer of surface enamel [27]. Therefore, in many cases, occlusal lesions develop slowly and do not cavitate, making lesion detection with conventional methods even more challenging than in the past. The hidden nature of occlusal caries makes diagnosis very subjective with visual inspection, where staining of the fissures can increase false positives and lead to unnecessary treatment. For occlusal lesions, tactile and visual inspection have been shown to have low sensitivity, ~0.3, because of the hidden nature of the lesions [28]. Tactile and visual inspection offer high specificity ~0.95 for advanced occlusal lesions that extend into the dentin, but the specificity is below 0.80 for lesions confined to the enamel that can be treated with non- surgical therapy [29]. The ability to detect near cavitated lesions is in itself problematic because the insertion of a sharp explorer can advance the progression of a lesion by damaging the outer surface of the lesion [30] and cause ingress of bacteria. Since conventional use of tactile assessment using a sharp explorer is no longer the gold standard for a clinical exam, teledentistry has potential to provide an evaluation close to the standard of care, with the exception of using tactile methods to feel the surface zone of smooth surface lesions [31]; however, these lesions are likely to be managed with topical therapies until obvious cavitation.

Optical caries detection systems have the potential to assist with visual assessment for the use of teledentistry. The list of systems on the market at the time of this article is extensive and expanding. Optical caries detection can be categorized as either scattering-based or fluorescence-based. The aim of this chapter is to not review all of these systems but highlight studies that are the most relevant to oral health evaluation in teledentistry. Most of these studies focused on assessing permanent teeth rather than primary teeth.

3.4 Scattering-Based Optical Scattering Detection Systems

Newer optical methods, such as the Midwest Caries ID™ (MID) and CP-OCT, have the potential to detect early non-cavitated occlusal lesions using non-ionizing, safe radiation (light). Increasing the accuracy of detecting and assessing early carious lesions with either objective direct measurements or an imaging modality that can allow remote assessment would serve children in critical communities. A potential objective caries detection measurement that could be collected by adjunct personnel may be accomplished using readings from the visible light based Midwest Caries

ID™ (Dentsply, York, PA) [32–34]. There is potential for adjunct personnel to electronically send a table of recorded readings from Midwest Caries ID™ to aid an offsite dentist in treatment planning.

Another emerging method for teledentistry includes near infrared imaging modalities, such as Cross-Polarization Optical Coherence Tomography (CP-OCT) [35, 36]. CP-OCT can be compared conceptually to ultrasound imaging since both techniques use an incident beam and measure a reflected or backscattered signal. Conventional OCT and the polarized enhanced CP-OCT has been shown to detect early carious lesions through an increase in light scattering [37–39]. CP-OCT is promising because it performs a real time optical image of the microstructure of the tissue, without radiation or surgical intervention [40]. Multiple OCT images can be produced within seconds, which is advantageous as a clinical detection technique [37]. The rapid acquisition of CP-OCT imaging can allow adjunct dental personnel to use the device for preventive dental screenings. Acquired CP-OCT images can later be interpreted by a dentist; however, there are few comparisons between other less costly optical devices, such as the Midwest Caries ID™ (MID) and simple visual camera images (CAM).

The MID uses a Light-Emitting Diode to emit a range of red light and then measures the scattering of light due to mineral changes experienced from carious lesions to determine if carious lesions exist [33, 34]. Red light normally scatters in sound tissue in a predominantly forward direction with minimal light being backscattered. As the mineral content of the measured area becomes less mineralized, more back scattering is detected, since demineralization causes isotropic (360°) scattering [41]. MID detects this increase in backscattering but there are few studies examining how much backscattering intensity is interpreted as caries. The individual measurements with the MID device occurred after calibration of the device. Teeth should be kept moist. The tip of the device can be inserted vertically on the surface of each tooth and moved around slightly (without pressure) in the pits and fissure area between the reference points. The MID uses a red indicator light to communicate to the examiner the presence of demineralization. In addition the MID produces sound at two frequencies; with the higher frequency designed to detect higher scattering being associated with a larger more extensive amount of decay (score = 2).

Both CP-OCT and MID (Fig. 3.1) do not have markedly superior diagnostic values from simple CAM assessment when assessing non-cavitated lesions (Table 3.2). These values were calculated from a gold standard of histology examination after sectioning [15]. It is important to keep in mind that, ICDAS-II score 1 and 2 teeth have both been shown to have demineralization extending into the dentin in approximately 17–33 % of *in vitro* cases [19, 42, 43]. Although MID and CP-OCT were useful in detecting the presence of demineralization, examiners were not able to utilize these devices to adequately assess the depth of the demineralization. The limitations of CP-OCT can be explained when examining Fig. 3.1. Demineralization caused the incident linearly polarized NIR light to be highly scattered and depolarized. The pit and fissure area near the reference point 'r1' (Fig. 3.2b, arrow) indicated extensive demineralization for E5 and E6 that was much greater than small surface demineralization; however, the scattering was so extensive in the upper

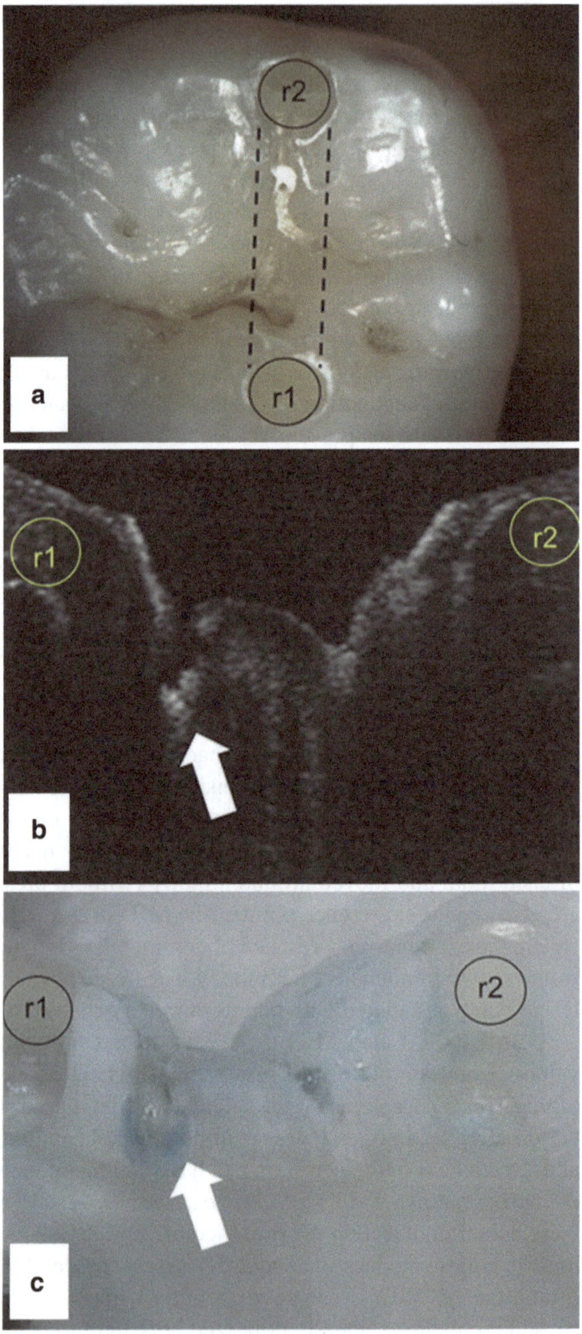

Fig. 3.1 Each tooth had two composite reference points (r1 and r2). The test area was the fissure area between the points. (**a**) All CAM images were assessed Score '2'. All MID Scorings were '0'. (**b**) CP-OCT images were taken before tooth sectioning. CP-OCT images are presented in grayscale. Black areas have low scattering and white areas have high scattering. All CP-OCT scorings were '2' based on the fissure area near r1 (*arrow*). (**c**) Histological evaluation using caries indicator dye confirmed demineralization extending into enamel and dentin with Score of '2'(*arrow*) (Picture from Van Hilsen et al., *BMC Oral Health*, 2012)

Table 3.2 Comparison between visual camera (CAM) based caries assessment and scattering based caries detection methods: Midwest Caries ID (MID) and CP-OCT

	Disease defined as score 1, 2		Disease defined as score 2		
	Sen	*Sp*	*Sen*	*Sp*	*ICC (95 % CI)*
CAM	80.5	52.5	48.0	57.8	0.75 (0.64–0.84)
MID	46.9	85.0	17.3	88.0	0.83 (0.75–0.90)
CP-OCT	83.4	45.0	44.2	72.7	0.49 (0.34–0.65)

Adapted from Van Hilsen, *BMC Oral Health* 2012

Mean Sensitivity (Sen) and Specificity (Sp) diagnostic values are shown from two examiners each making two separate assessments spaced 1–2 weeks apart. Diagnostic values are reported at two disease thresholds defined after histological sectioning. Mean values of the Sen and Sp are reported. The Intraclass Correlation Coefficient (ICC) represents the absolute agreement of all four examinations for each diagnostic method. 95 % Confidence Intervals are presented

portion of the lesion that the full extent of the demineralization was not measured by CP-OCT. This was likely because the scattering degraded and attenuated the incident light. The CP-OCT NIR light could not penetrate deep enough through the entire lesion. This observation agrees with past studies where demineralization in enamel hides the underlying tooth structure [44, 45]. It is important to point out that although the intensity of the incident light and the sensitivity of the CP-OCT detector can be increased in the future, improving these factors may not be able to markedly improve signal penetration, especially at intensity levels that are safe for diagnostic CP-OCT imaging.

Another limitation in CP-OCT imaging was that it was difficult to assess the fissure depth in reference to the DEJ. The DEJ was not apparent in the majority of the images of this study. This was likely caused from the internal reflection angle (critical angle) of light traveling through enamel back to the detector. To clarify, as the returning (back-scattered) signal traveled back through the enamel toward the tooth surface, the signal could be internally reflected when the occlusal topography angles were greater than 37–54° to incident plane (the range is dependent on the water moisture level). In certain occlusal samples, internal reflection could attenuate the backscattered signal from deeper enamel and dentin layers from returning to the CP-OCT for measurement. Another explanation is that the CP-OCT system could not actively focus well below the surface to acquire the deeper DEJ signal; however, the low numerical aperture lens on the probe was designed to capture deeper signals.

To assess examiner agreement and reliability when assessing sound versus any demineralization (score 0 versus 1, 2), the Intraclass Correlation Coefficient (ICC) was calculated for each of these methods (Table 3.2). This ICC value represents an agreement of four readings: two examiners each making two separate assessments spaced 1–2 weeks apart. MID was found to have the highest ICC, and the overall CP-OCT ICC indicated that there was high variability in assessing the images. This highlights an important and often overlooked assessment of caries detection used in teledentistry. Reliability in caries assessment is crucial, and CP-OCT requires a highly skilled and trained evaluator.

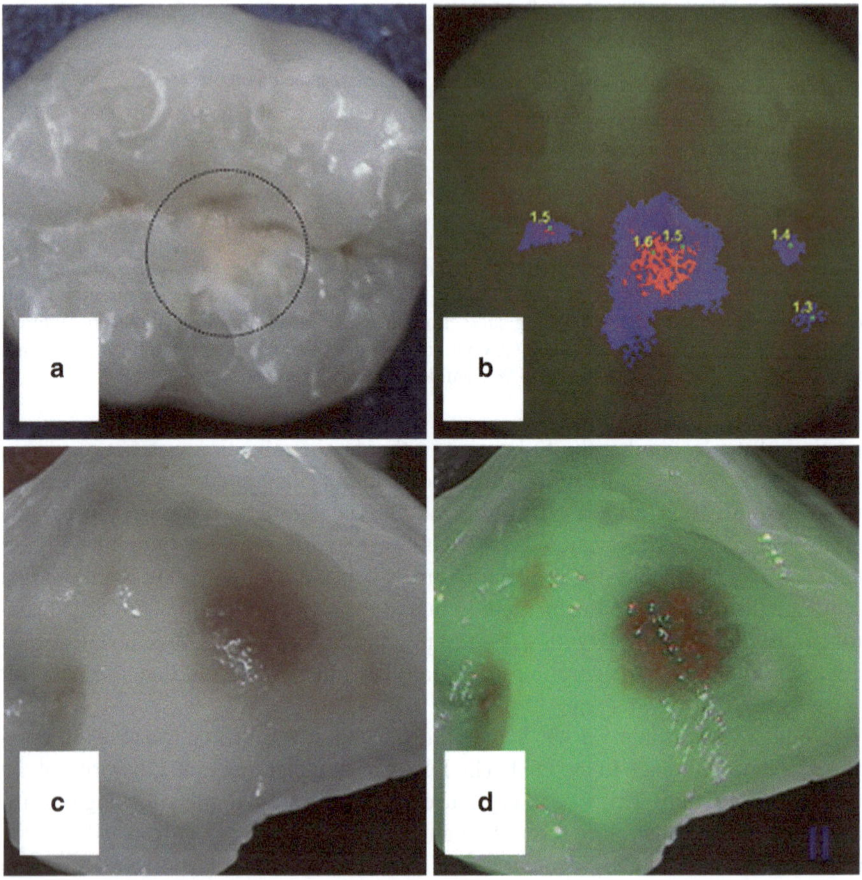

Fig. 3.2 (**a**) Visual image (CAM) of an extracted tooth with a lesion that did not penetrate past the DEJ (Teledentistry lesion score = 1). (**b**) The *fluorescence-based* imaging (Spectra/VistaProof®) illuminates the tooth with 405 nm light and quantifies the degree of fluorescence emitted with a false color scale. (**c**) Perioperative images of a tooth after the majority of dentinal caries were removed. Stained dentin remained. (**d**) *Fluorescence-based* imaging (Soprolife®) illuminates the tooth with 450 nm light and the green and red shifted fluorescence is visualized. The red shift fluorescence correlates strongly with the visual brown staining seen in (**c**). All analysis was done soon after extraction to preserve porphyrins concentration within the tooth (Images from author)

3.5 Fluorescence-Based Optical Detection Systems

Fluorescence-based detection systems have been extensively studied and used in clinical practice. Common examples are the Diagnodent® (KaVo Dental, Lake Zurich, IL, USA), the Soprolife® intraoral fluorescence camera (Acteon, La Ciotat, France), the VistaProof® intraoral fluorescence camera (Dürr Dental, Bietigheim-Bissingen, Germany) which is marketed in the U.S. as the Spectra® Caries detection system (Air Techniques, Melville, NY). Each of these systems share a similar mechanism in that the system illuminates the tooth with a LED light source, albeit each with a distinct wavelength, and detects re-emitted light at a longer wavelength with lower energy. The detected fluorescent signal is not generated from sound dental tissue but from porphyrins, synthesized by bacteria, which populate a carious lesion [46]. Thus, it is not a change in the tissue structure or depth that is directly related to the signal, rather the volume concentration of porphyrins. In addition, porphyrins are not significantly produced by cariogenic Bacteria. They are produced by other co-populating bacteria [47]. These are the likely reasons that enamel lesions are detected by the Diagnodent® with very low sensitivity (~0.4) [48]. Early white spot lesions with no bacteria involvement do not produce a fluorescence signal above the background sound enamel since these lesions lack porphyrin metabolites [49]. The SoproLife® and Spectra/VistaProof® system have been evaluated in the context of differentiating non-cavitated lesions versus cavitated occlusal lesions [20, 50]. In that evaluation, the sensitivity of the assessment was similar to an visual image (92–95 %) that could be used in teledentistry [20]. The specificity of these intraoral fluorescence (37–55 %) were no higher than visual assessment (63 %) [20].

There is growing effort to connect their diagnostic evaluation with treatment decisions [16]. The author encourages the simple use of the Teledentistry Lesion Scale (TLS) in evaluating future systems, although expanded scoring does help initially establish the cut-off values in establishing receiver operator curves ('sensitivity' and '1-specificity' values plotted at different threshold values) [51], which is needed prior to teledentistry based evaluation.

There is concern that assessment of fluorescence-based imaging (Spectra/VistaProof®) can overestimate the number of individuals who have occlusal enamel and dentinal caries at distinct cut-off fluorescence values [52]. This means that assessment of these fluorescence images had a low positive predictive value, which takes into account the measured sensitivity, specificity, and overall disease prevalence. In other words, most teeth that were 'assessed as carious' were sound. In a teledentistry application, this can lead to the over use of referral for unnecessary treatment and not solely utilizing prevention and CAMBRA based topical management. Importantly, assessing fluorescence-based (Spectra/VistaProof®) imaging was found to have a remarkably high negative predictive value (NPV) for enamel and dentinal lesions (93–98 %) [52]. This means that most teeth that were 'assessed as sound' were sound. The aforementioned study did not histologically validate non-cavitated lesions unless there were visual signs of lesion activity, and this may be one reason that the study reported a high NPV. The importance is that a caries detection system with a high NPV (even if it has a low PPV) can be used in teledentistry to 'rule out' a patient as having decay and can aid in the appropriate management of the patient.

There are new opportunities in teledentistry to use diagnostic imaging during the perioperative and post-operative surgical procedure for midlevel providers such as dental therapists. This idea is in its infancy (especially in the United States where dental therapists only practice in Alaska and Minnesota), but diagnostic imaging could be used to remotely assess the caries removal process and help evaluate the performance of these midlevel providers. Fluorescence-based imaging has potential to assess the degree of dentinal caries [53, 54]. Preliminary evaluation by the author has seen a high correlation between visual staining and fluorescent based imaging assessment (Fig. 3.2c, d). This is reminiscent of how fluorescence-based imaging may not outperform visual image assessment for initial treatment planning. Future studies are needed to investigate this potential use in teledentistry.

3.6 Summary

Despite considerable advancements in the technology of early caries detection, advanced imaging and detection methods have not been shown to have markedly superior diagnostic values from simple visual image analysis for use in teledentistry.

References

1. Featherstone JDB, Doméjean S. Minimal intervention dentistry: part 1. From "compulsive" restorative dentistry to rational therapeutic strategies. Br Dent J. 2012;213:441–5.
2. American Academy of Pediatric Dentistry; American Academy of Pediatrics; American Academy of Pediatric Dentistry Council on Clinical Affairs. Policy on early childhood caries (ECC): classifications, consequences, and preventive strategies. Pediatr Dent. 2005–2006;27(7 Suppl):31–3.
3. Hale KJ. Oral health risk assessment timing and establishment of the dental home. Pediatrics. 2003;111(5 Pt 1):1113–6.
4. Kopycka-Kedzierawski DT, Bell CH, Billings RJ. Prevalence of dental caries in Early Head Start children as diagnosed using teledentistry. Pediatr Dent. 2008;30:329–33.
5. Yoon RK, Smaldone AM, Edelstein BL. Early childhood caries screening tools: a comparison of four approaches. J Am Dent Assoc. 2012;143:756–63.
6. Featherstone JDB, White JM, Hoover CI, Rapozo-Hilo M, Weintraub JA, Wilson RS, Zhan L, Gansky SA. A randomized clinical trial of anticaries therapies targeted according to risk assessment (caries management by risk assessment). Caries Res. 2012;46:118–29.
7. Gao X, Di Wu I, Lo ECM, Chu CH, Hsu C-YS, Wong MCM. Validity of caries risk assessment programmes in preschool children. J Dent. 2013;41:787–95.
8. Rugg-Gunn AJ, Do L. Effectiveness of water fluoridation in caries prevention. Community Dent Oral Epidemiol. 2012;40 Suppl 2:55–64.
9. American Academy on Pediatric Dentistry Council on Clinical Affairs. Policy on use of a caries-risk assessment tool (CAT) for infants, children, and adolescents. Pediatr Dent. 2008–2009;30(7 Suppl):29–33.
10. Crall JJ. Rethinking prevention. Pediatr Dent. 2006;28:96–101; discussion 192–8.
11. Tsang P, Qi F, Shi W. Medical approach to dental caries: fight the disease, not the lesion. Pediatr Dent. 2006;28:188–91; discussion 192–8.
12. Steiner M, Helfenstein U, Marthaler TM. Dental predictors of high caries increment in children. J Dent Res. 1992;71:1926–33.
13. Ramos-Gomez F, Ng MW. Into the future: keeping healthy teeth caries free: pediatric CAMBRA protocols. J Calif Dent Assoc. 2011;39:723–33.
14. Heller KE, Reed SG, Bruner FW, Eklund SA, Burt BA. Longitudinal evaluation of sealing molars with and without incipient dental caries in a public health program. J Public Health Dent. 1995;55:148–53.

15. Van Hilsen Z, Jones RS. Comparing potential early caries assessment methods for teledentistry. BMC Oral Health. 2013;13:16.
16. Tassery H, Levallois B, Terrer E, Manton DJ, Otsuki M, Koubi S, Gugnani N, Panayotov I, Jacquot B, Cuisinier F, Rechmann P. Use of new minimum intervention dentistry technologies in caries management. Aust Dent J. 2013;58 Suppl 1:40–59.
17. Mitropoulos P, Rahiotis C, Stamatakis H, Kakaboura A. Diagnostic performance of the visual caries classification system ICDAS II versus radiography and micro-computed tomography for proximal caries detection: an in vitro study. J Dent. 2010;38:859–67.
18. ICDASII. Rationale and evidence for the international caries detection and assessment system (ICDASII). 2005.
19. Diniz MB, Rodrigues JA, Hug I, Cordeiro Rde C, Lussi A. Reproducibility and accuracy of the ICDAS-II for occlusal caries detection. Community Dent Oral Epidemiol. 2009;37:399–404.
20. Rechmann P, Charland D, Rechmann BMT, Featherstone JDB. Performance of laser fluorescence devices and visual examination for the detection of occlusal caries in permanent molars. J Biomed Opt. 2012;17:036006.
21. Jablonski-Momeni A, Stucke J, Steinberg T, Heinzel-Gutenbrunner M. Use of ICDAS-II, fluorescence-based methods, and radiography in detection and treatment decision of occlusal caries lesions: an in vitro study. Int J Dent. 2012;2012:371595.
22. Diniz MB, Lima LM, Eckert G, Zandona AG, Cordeiro RC, Pinto LS. In vitro evaluation of ICDAS and radiographic examination of occlusal surfaces and their association with treatment decisions. Oper Dent. 2011;36:133–42.
23. Ramos-Gomez FJ, Crystal YO, Domejean S, Featherstone JDB. Minimal intervention dentistry: part 3. Paediatric dental care – prevention and management protocols using caries risk assessment for infants and young children. Br Dent J. 2012;213:501–8.
24. Domejean S, White JM, Featherstone JD. Validation of the CDA CAMBRA caries risk assessment–a six-year retrospective study. J Calif Dent Assoc. 2011;39:709–15.
25. Guerrieri A, Gaucher C, Bonte E, Lasfargues JJ. Minimal intervention dentistry: part 4. Detection and diagnosis of initial caries lesions. Br Dent J. 2012;213:551–7.
26. Brown LJ, Kaste LM, Selwitz RH, Furman LJ. Dental caries and sealant usage in U.S. children, 1988–1991: selected findings from the Third National Health and Nutrition Examination Survey. J Am Dent Assoc. 1996;127:335–43.
27. Pitts NB. Diagnostic tools and measurements–impact on appropriate care. Community Dent Oral Epidemiol. 1997;25:24–35.
28. Ten Cate JM, van Amerongen AJ. Caries diagnosis: conventional methods. In: Early detection of dental caries. Indianapolis: Indiana University; 1996.
29. Bader JD, Shugars DA, Bonito AJ. Systematic reviews of selected dental caries diagnostic and management methods. J Dent Educ. 2001;65:960–8.
30. Ekstrand KR, Ricketts DN, Kidd EA. Reproducibility and accuracy of three methods for assessment of demineralization depth of the occlusal surface: an in vitro examination. Caries Res. 1997;31:224–31.
31. Nyvad B, Machiulskiene V, Baelum V. Reliability of a new caries diagnostic system differentiating between active and inactive caries lesions. Caries Res. 1999;33:252–60.
32. Rodrigues JA, Hug I, Neuhaus KW, Lussi A. Light-emitting diode and laser fluorescence-based devices in detecting occlusal caries. J Biomed Opt. 2011;16:107003.
33. Hastar E, Yildiz E, Aktan AM. The effect of fissure sealants on the values of two different caries detection devices. Photomed Laser Surg. 2012;30:683–7.
34. Aktan AM, Cebe MA, Ciftci ME, Sirin Karaarslan E. A novel LED-based device for occlusal caries detection. Lasers Med Sci. 2012;27:1157–63.
35. Fried D, Xie J, Shafi S, Featherstone JDB, Breunig T, Lee CQ. Early detection of dental caries and lesion progression with polarization sensitive optical coherence tomography. J Biomed Optics. 2002;7:618–27.

36. Staninec M, Douglas SM, Darling CL, Chan K, Kang H, Lee RC, Fried D. Non-destructive clinical assessment of occlusal caries lesions using near-IR imaging methods. Lasers Surg Med. 2011;43:951–9.
37. Shimada Y, Sadr A, Burrow MF, Tagami J, Ozawa N, Sumi Y. Validation of swept-source optical coherence tomography (SS-OCT) for the diagnosis of occlusal caries. J Dent. 2010;38:655–65.
38. Hobin K, Jiao JJ, Chulsung L, Le MH, Darling CL, Fried DL. Nondestructive assessment of early tooth demineralization using cross-polarization optical coherence tomography. IEEE J Sel Top Quantum Electron. 2010;16:870–6.
39. Holtzman JS, Osann K, Pharar J, Lee K, Ahn Y, Tucker T, Sabet S, Chen Z, Gukasyan R, Wilder-Smith P. Ability of optical coherence tomography to detect caries beneath commonly used dental sealants. Lasers Surg Med. 2010;42:752–9.
40. Huang D, Swanson EA, Lin CP, Schuman JS, Stinson WG, Chang W, Hee MR, Flotte T, Gregory K, Puliafito CA, Fujimoto JG. Optical coherence tomography. Science. 1991;254:1178–81.
41. Darling CL, Huynh GD, Fried D. Light scattering properties of natural and artificially demineralized dental enamel at 1310 nm. J Biomed Opt. 2006;11:34011–23.
42. Jablonski-Momeni A, Stachniss V, Ricketts DN, Heinzel-Gutenbrunner M, Pieper K. Reproducibility and accuracy of the ICDAS-II for detection of occlusal caries in vitro. Caries Res. 2008;42:79–87.
43. Ekstrand KR, Martignon S, Ricketts DJ, Qvist V. Detection and activity assessment of primary coronal caries lesions: a methodologic study. Oper Dent. 2007;32:225–35.
44. Baumgartner A, Hitzenberger CK, Sattmann H, Robi B, Moritz A, Sperr W, Fercher AF. Polarization-sensitive optical coherence tomography of dental structures. Caries Res. 2000;34:59–69.
45. Chen Y, Otis L, Piao D, Zhu Q. Characterization of dentin, enamel, and carious lesions by a polarization-sensitive optical coherence tomography system. Appl Opt. 2005;44:2041–8.
46. Koenig K, Schneckenburger H, Hemmer J, Tromberg BJ, Steiner RW. In-vivo fluorescence detection and imaging of porphyrin-producing bacteria in the human skin and in the oral cavity for diagnosis of acne vulgaris, caries, and squamous cell carcinoma. Proc. SPIE 2135, Advances in Laser and Light Spectroscopy to Diagnose Cancer and Other Diseases. 1994;2135:129–38.
47. Lennon AM, Buchalla W, Brune L, Zimmermann O, Gross U, Attin T. The ability of selected oral microorganisms to emit red fluorescence. Caries Res. 2006;40:2–5.
48. Shi XQ, Welander U, Angmar-Månsson B. Occlusal caries detection with KaVo DIAGNOdent and radiography: an in vitro comparison. Caries Res. 2000;34:151–8.
49. Lussi A, Megert B, Longbottom C, Reich E, Francescut P. Clinical performance of a laser fluorescence device for detection of occlusal caries lesions. Eur J Oral Sci. 2001;109:14–9.
50. Diniz MB, Boldieri T, Rodrigues JA, Santos-Pinto L, Lussi A, Cordeiro RCL. The performance of conventional and fluorescence-based methods for occlusal caries detection: an in vivo study with histologic validation. J Am Dent Assoc. 2012;143:339–50.
51. Christenson RH. Evidence-based laboratory medicine – a guide for critical evaluation of in vitro laboratory testing. Ann Clin Biochem. 2007;44(Pt 2):111–30.
52. Jablonski-Momeni A, Heinzel-Gutenbrunner M, Klein SMC. In vivo performance of the VistaProof fluorescence-based camera for detection of occlusal lesions. Clin Oral Invest. 2013. [Published ahead of print].
53. Ganter P, Al-Ahmad A, Wrbas K-T, Hellwig E, Altenburger M. The use of computer-assisted FACE for minimal-invasive caries excavation. Clin Oral Invest. 2014;18:745–51.
54. Stoll R, Urban-Klein B, Giacomin P, Loukas A, Jablonski-Momeni A. In vivo assessment of caries excavation with a fluorescence camera compared to direct bacteriological sampling and quantitative analysis using flow cytometry. Lasers Med Sci. 2013. [Published ahead of print]

Chapter 4
Home Telecare Program on Oral Health

Hon K. Yuen

Abstract This chapter describes the use of interactive videoconferencing as a strategy for oral hygiene training which may lead to a change in oral hygiene service delivery methods, an improvement in access to quality oral health care, and a reduction in oral disease burden on underserved populations. Clients who may benefit most from the oral home telecare are those who demonstrate cognitive impairment and/or physical disabilities, especially upper extremity dysfunction with manual dexterity impairment, and/or orofacial dysfunction. Preventive oral homecare via videoconferencing has been shown to build long-term habits for maintaining oral hygiene among people with chronic medical conditions or disabilities, thereby maintaining the continuity of care with conventional dental care services. Oral home telecare educational and training services provided by occupational therapists can be integrated into a broader, interdisciplinary, comprehensive telerehabilitation delivery program to enhance the patient's general health and overall quality of life.

Keywords Home telecare • Telerehabilitation • Oral care • Dental health education • Adaptive devices • Videoconferencing • Technology

4.1 What Is Oral Home Telecare?

Oral home telecare, a term coined by Tomuro [1], is defined as "a care services system based on interactive motion-picture transmission between households and healthcare providers" (p.165).

H.K. Yuen, PhD, OTR/L
Department of Occupational Therapy, School of Health Professions,
University of Alabama at Birmingham, 1720 Second Avenue South,
Birmingham, AL 35294, USA
e-mail: yuen@uab.edu

S. Kumar (ed.), *Teledentistry*, Health Informatics,
DOI 10.1007/978-3-319-08973-7_4

4.2 Evolution of Oral Home Telecare

A pioneer study on oral home telecare was conducted by Tomuro in Japan [1]. Through videophone, Tomuro provided real-time live interactive oral care training embedded in general health care education to four community-dwelling elderly men with brain damage; three of them had hemiplegia and aphasia [1, 2]. The oral home telecare was conducted between a dental health professional and the elders and their spouses for about 30 min once a week with a median of 10.5 weeks. Analysis of the changes in oral health among the four elders at post-telecare training indicated an improvement in independence of their oral homecare skills, specifically toothbrushing, mouth rinsing and denture wearing, and a reduction in dental plaque scores.

Based on the oral home telecare concept proposed by Tomuro [1, 2], Yuen and Pope [3] conducted a case study on two women with quadriplegia in the United States to test the feasibility of delivering oral hygiene training using assistive oral hygiene devices via computer-based, real-time interactive videoconferencing. The study also explored the acceptability of the oral home telecare services to the clients. Results indicated that it was feasible to provide oral home telecare training via videoconferencing for these two adults with quadriplegia, and both participants were satisfied with the oral home telecare services and enthusiastic about using the services.

Extending this feasibility study, Yuen [4] conducted a small pilot trial (one group pre- and post-test design with a 9-month post-training longitudinal follow-up) to evaluate the effectiveness of an oral home telecare program in the use of assistive oral hygiene devices to improve gingival health among eight adults with quadriplegia, and to investigate the impact of their oral home telecare experience. Individualized training was conducted on an average of five 15–30 min sessions across 12 weeks between each adult with quadriplegia and an occupational therapist (a rehabilitation specialist) with collaboration from a dental hygienist using PC-based, high-speed, two-way, real-time interactive videoconferencing. Gingival health assessment using the Löe-Silness gingival index (LSGI) was conducted at baseline, 6 months, and 12 months.

At 1-year follow-up, participants showed significant improvement in their LSGI scores with less gingival inflammation. Participants also completed a 21-item questionnaire, the Oral Home Telecare Questionnaire (see Table 4.1) [3, 4], which is used to measure participants' satisfaction with the quality of oral care and interaction with the therapist via videoconferencing. Consistent with the results of reduction in gingival inflammation, participants rated improvement in their oral health care and the interaction with the therapist being highly satisfied.

In the area of oral hygiene behaviors, an increase in the frequency of daily toothbrushing, dental flossing and the use of an oral irrigator 6 months from baseline was reported, and the same frequency of oral hygiene was maintained at 12 months. In addition, participants brushed their teeth longer during their toothbrushing demonstration at 6- and 12-month assessments. Yuen [4] concluded that an average of five sessions of videoconferencing across 12 weeks of oral hygiene training in the use of adaptive oral hygiene devices was sufficient to increase participants' oral hygiene frequency and use of adaptive devices. This resulted in a significant reduction of gingival inflammation and the establishment of long-term oral hygiene habits.

In-depth interviews immediately after the 12-week oral home telecare program indicated that participants felt more aware of their oral health and made a more

Table 4.1 Oral Home Telecare Questionnaire (OHTQ)

Item #	Item
1	I can always trust the videoconferencing equipment to work
2	Video visits are a convenient form of dental healthcare for me
3	There were technical problems that made it difficult for me to hear or see the therapist[a]
4	The therapist can get a good understanding of my oral hygiene condition over the videoconferencing
5	The home telecare helps me to better manage my oral health needs
6	Using videoconferencing the therapist will be able to monitor my oral health condition well
7	The use of the videoconferencing equipment seems difficult to me[a]
8	I would recommend oral home telecare to a friend
9	I got enough information via oral home telecare to perform oral hygiene
10	I felt comfortable with the videoconferencing equipment used relative to in-person
11	I can explain my mouth and tooth care problems well enough during a video visit
12	I can be as satisfied talking to the therapist over videoconferencing as talking in person
13	The lack of physical contact during a video visit is not a problem
14	Oral home telecare can save my time for visiting the therapist
15	Video visits make it easier for me to contact the therapist
16	I would be willing to use oral home telecare again
17	I feel more control over my oral health care since using oral home telecare
18	I am more involved in my oral health care since using home telecare
19	I have become more active in my oral health care since using oral home telecare
20	My oral health is better than it was before I joined the home telecare
21	Oral home telecare violates my privacy[a]

Note: Each item is rated on a 5-point Likert-type scale, where 1 = strongly disagree, 2 = disagree, 3 = neutral, 4 = agree, 5 = strongly agree

[a]Items are worded negatively and need to be recoded

Oral Home Telecare Questionnaire (OHTQ) is adapted from the Telemedicine Satisfaction and Usefulness Questionnaire and the Telemedicine Perception Questionnaire [5, 6]. The internal consistency reliability of the OHTQ estimated by Cronbach's alpha was .87 [4]

conscientious effort to perform their oral hygiene. Participants generally accepted the new technology (i.e., videoconferencing) and were enthusiastic about having the opportunity to receive oral home telecare educational services. Participants commented that the oral home telecare service was convenient as it was conducted at their home without traveling to a clinic. Few participants had concerns about loss of privacy via videoconferencing. Participants who never had videoconferencing experience felt a little embarrassed or strange during the first encounter with the therapist, but they quickly became used to the therapist looking and talking to them on the screen.

4.3 Types of Clients Who May Benefit from Oral Home Telecare

Based on the literature [1–4], clients who may benefit most from the oral home telecare are those who demonstrate cognitive impairment and/or physical disabilities, especially upper extremity dysfunction with manual dexterity impairment. For example, clients with brain damage who exhibit hemiparesis and cognitive impairment, and clients with an incomplete injury of the cervical spinal cord segments (i.e., quadriplegia) who have difficulty manipulating a manual toothbrush or dental floss to perform oral hygiene but do not totally depend on others to complete the task. Other vulnerable populations that may benefit from the oral home telecare services include patients with chronic medical conditions such as systemic sclerosis, in which manual dexterity impairments and orofacial dysfunction (e.g., microstomia/small mouth and xerostomia/dry mouth) may complicate oral hygiene and lead to oral health problems [7–9]. Hand deformity and limited oral aperture may affect oral hygiene performance as well as willingness to perform oral hygiene [7, 10]. Patients may require an adaptive oral hygiene device due to small mouth opening, and need to perform mouth stretching exercises to increase the size of their oral aperture.

The goal of the oral home telecare program is to improve oral hygiene so as to prevent severe oral diseases such as caries and periodontal disease. The program cannot reverse any existing oral disease condition. Therefore, patients who are likely to benefit most from the program are those who have recently received comprehensive dental cleaning and treatment, or those who were recently injured or diagnosed, and need to learn a new set of skills to maintain their oral hygiene, including exercises that can improve their orofacial and manual dexterity function. Some of these patients are home-bound, have limited mobility, and/or use a wheelchair which may impose physical barriers to accessing dental care. Oral home telecare provides an avenue to decrease physical barriers and improve access to oral health care.

Due to the nature of their impairments and disabilities, these patients may require special adaptation of commercially available oral hygiene devices, labor-intensive training in the use of adaptive oral hygiene devices, training on correct performance of mouth stretching exercises, and repeated positive reinforcement to assist in establishing regular mouth stretching exercises and oral hygiene habits. For patients without upper extremity impairment, orofacial dysfunction, or cognitive impairment, this kind of intensive training (i.e., oral home telecare services) is not required. Instead, other avenues for receiving oral health information and training via the Internet, as reported in the literature [11, 12], may be sufficient.

4.4 Health Care Professionals Who Are Qualified to Provide Oral Home Telecare

Given the type of patients who may benefit from oral home telecare services, an ideal health care provider team should consist of a dental hygienist and an occupational therapist. Occupational therapists are rehabilitation professionals who specialize in enabling people with disabilities to participate activities of daily living (ADL) such as self-care or personal hygiene in their desired roles, context, and life situations [13]. Within their scope of practice, occupational therapists incorporate several approaches to enhance patient safety and independence in performing various self-care activities. These therapeutic approaches include remediation, education, compensation, modification, and adaptation.

Based on the patient's physical and/or cognitive ability to manipulate oral hygiene devices, their preference for the device, recommendations from the dental hygienist, as well as input from the caregiver, if applicable, the occupational therapist may recommend to the patient appropriate oral hygiene devices such as powered toothbrushes, interdental cleaning devices with elongated and enlarged handles, as well as universal cuffs so that the device can be easily held with minimal hand dexterity. The occupational therapist may suggest adaptive strategies to perform oral hygiene and/or appropriate setup to facilitate performance of oral hygiene routines.

One of the merits of having occupational therapists provide oral home telecare services is that their education and training to the patient can be integrated into a broader, interdisciplinary, comprehensive telerehabilitation delivery program to enhance the patient's general health and overall quality of life. Such services can be reimbursed. Based on the results of a payment practice survey for telerehabilitation conducted in 2002, at least four states' Medicaid programs provided reimbursement for occupational therapy telerehabilitation services at that time [11]. With the continued expansion of Medicaid and private insurance reimbursement for telemedicine services to more states [14], reimbursement for telerehabilitation, including oral home telecare services, will be more prevalent.

4.5 Oral Home Telecare Intervention

Between the two team members/providers, typically, the dental hygienist (in the presence of the occupational therapist) is responsible for educating patients and caregivers (if applicable/available) about dental health during the first two sessions. The occupational therapist is responsible for (1) recommending oral hygiene devices and adaptive devices such as universal cuffs, (2) training in the proper way to use the adaptive oral hygiene device, (3) motivating the patient and increasing their self-efficacy to complete daily oral hygiene, and (4) teaching and monitoring the patient in the completion of daily mouth stretching exercises, if applicable [13].

As a complement to the work of dental hygienists, occupational therapists have traditionally employed activity analysis, behavioral and cognitive-behavioral principles to enhance patients' compliance with oral hygiene and/or mouth stretching exercises. Strategies may include motivational interviews, demonstration, modeling, and return demonstration on the proper use of the adaptive device to perform oral hygiene [15]. During these training sessions, supervised practice of oral hygiene, and provision of immediate corrective feedback and positive reinforcement in the use of adaptive oral hygiene devices correctly, safely, independently and efficiently to complete oral hygiene is emphasized. Patient skill demonstration and feedback on oral hygiene performance are especially important for persons with disabilities during oral care education and training [16, 17]. Modification of the environment, set up, and the adaptive devices will be continued throughout the first few sessions to ensure optimum independence in using the oral hygiene devices to complete oral hygiene routines. Coaching a caregiver, attendant or co-habitant, if available, to improve the patient's oral hygiene performance is essential. A home visit by the occupational therapist may be required to set up the appropriate environment or add modifications to the oral hygiene device.

Through problem-solving with the therapist, patients may come up with strategies to address difficulties that they encountered in using oral hygiene devices. In Yuen's study [4], four participants with quadriplegia came up with ideas and solutions to help improve their oral hygiene performance, which included obtaining a new cuff to secure the oral hygiene device on the hand, exploring the option of a new waterpik system that hooks to the shower head so the participant could use it in the shower, creatively applying a piece of Dycem® (an anti-slip sheet) to secure the oral hygiene device, and designing a custom-made perpendicular dowel to turn an electric toothbrush on/off with the other hand. The therapist reinforces such strategy use, and provides ongoing support. Finally, through guidance from the therapist, the patient will come up a plan to sustain the oral hygiene habits.

Oral home telecare requires labor-intensive repeated training to patients on the handling skills involved in the use of assistive oral hygiene devices, repeated positive reinforcement to motivate their compliance with recommended oral hygiene practice or mouth stretching exercises, and monitoring and assistance in establishing regular oral hygiene habits. Provision of continual motivation and training in the use of adaptive oral hygiene devices cannot be completed in one or two sessions during regular dental clinic visits. In addition, patients may not be able to learn and remember all the instructions in a few sessions.

Oral home telecare education and training is by no means a replacement for traditional dental visits with cleaning and education from dental health professionals. However, it is well documented that patient education at routine dental visits is not sufficient to motivate an individual to maintain oral hygiene routines [17]. Preventive oral homecare via videoconferencing has been shown to build long-term habits for maintaining oral hygiene among people with quadriplegia, thereby maintaining the continuity of care with conventional dental care services [4].

However, oral home telecare can serve as a substitute or supplement to face-to-face approaches for in-home therapy visits. Such mode of care can reduce costs (time and travel distance), and extend limited available professional personnel to serve widely distributed geographic areas including rural/remote or underserved urban areas. Oral home telecare offers strategies to decrease physical barriers and communication difficulties and has been shown to improve the quality of dental health services for people with chronic medical conditions or disabilities [1, 4].

4.6 Future Directions

Building on the evidence from previous feasibility and pilot studies [1–4], a logical extension to validate the efficacy of oral care telecare training is to implement a multi-site, large-scale randomized clinical trial with a well-designed protocol. The core of the protocol should be applicable to a range of patients with cognitive and/or physical (upper extremity, manual dexterity, or orofacial) dysfunction. In terms of dissemination, the next step is to expand oral home telecare services by integrating them into the routine rehabilitation service delivery mechanism for people with chronic medical conditions or disabilities, with the ultimate goal of enhancing the quality of oral health care and reducing oral health access disparities among these at-risk populations.

With the birth of smart mobile devices, videoconferencing equipment such as videophone becomes obsolete. There are free videoconferencing software programs (e.g., Skype™ and *ooVoo*™) that can be downloaded from the Internet to the smart mobile device for use. It is expected that as the technology continues to improve, issues such as accessibility, technical challenges, privacy and security concerns that we face today will not be critical issues when delivering oral home telecare services in 5 or 10 years. However, reimbursement and licensure and/or medicolegal issues such as liability coverage, may be the real impediment to the wider implementation of oral home telecare services.

4.7 Conclusion

The use of interactive videoconferencing as a strategy for oral hygiene training may lead to a change in oral hygiene service delivery methods, an improvement in access to quality oral health care, and a reduction in oral disease burden on underserved populations. The public health impact of implementing oral home telecare is to extend access of preventive dental care to people with chronic medical conditions or disabilities who historically receive inadequate dental hygiene training, as well as to provide appropriate oral hygiene services delivery to geographically dispersed populations.

References

1. Tomuro K. Oral home telecare tutorials for the community-dwelling elderly. J Med Dent Sci. 2004;51(3):165–71.
2. Tomuro K. Development of oral home telecare programme for the home-dwelling elderly: a pilot study. Gerodontology. 2004;21(3):177–80.
3. Yuen HK, Pope C. Oral home telecare for adults with tetraplegia: a feasibility study. Spec Care Dentist. 2009;29(5):204–9.
4. Yuen HK. Effect of a home telecare program on oral health among adults with tetraplegia: a pilot study. Spinal Cord. 2013;51(6):477–81.
5. Bakken S, Grullon-Figueroa L, Izquierdo R, Lee NJ, Morin P, Palmas W, et al., IDEATel Consortium. Development, validation, and use of English and Spanish versions of the telemedicine satisfaction and usefulness questionnaire. J Am Med Inform Assoc. 2006;13(6):660–7.
6. Demiris G, Speedie S, Finkelstein S. A questionnaire for the assessment of patients' impressions of the risks and benefits of home telecare. J Telemed Telecare. 2000;6(5):278–84.
7. Poole JL, Brewer C, Rossie K, Good CC, Conte C, Steen V. Factors related to oral hygiene in persons with scleroderma. Int J Dent Hyg. 2005;3(1):13–7.

8. Scardina GA, Messina P. Systemic sclerosis: description and diagnostic role of the oral phenomena. Gen Dent. 2004;52(1):42–7.
9. Yuen H, Weng Y, Reed S, Summerlin L, Silver R. Factors associated with gingival inflammation among adults with systemic sclerosis. Int J Dent Hyg. 2014;12(1):55–61.
10. Kelsey JL, Lamster IB. Influence of musculoskeletal conditions on oral health among older adults. Am J Public Health. 2008;98(7):1177–83.
11. Chestnutt IG. The nature and quality of periodontal related patient information on the world-wide web. Br Dent J. 2002;193(11):657–9; discussion 643.
12. Ojima M, Hanioka T, Kuboniwa M, Nagata H, Shizukuishi S. Development of Web-based intervention system for periodontal health: a pilot study in the workplace. Med Inform Internet Med. 2003;28(4):291–8.
13. American Occupational Therapy Association. Scope of practice. Am J Occup. 2004;58:5.
14. Whitten P, Buis L. Private payer reimbursement for telemedicine services in the United States. Telemed J E Health. 2007;13(1):15–23.
15. Bellomo F, de Preux F, Chung J-P, Julien N, Budtz-Jorgensen E, Muller F. The advantages of occupational therapy in oral hygiene measures for institutionalised elderly adults. Gerodontology. 2005;22(1):8.
16. Milgrom P, Weinstein P, Chapko M, Grembowski D, Spadafora A. Dentists' attitudes and behaviors in counseling patients about oral self care. J Am Coll Dent. 1988;55(1):48–53.
17. Weinstein P, Milgrom P, Melnick S, Beach B, Spadafora A. How effective is oral hygiene instruction? Results after 6 and 24 weeks. J Public Health Dent. 1989;49(1):32–8.

Chapter 5
Teledentistry-Assisted Affiliated Practice Dental Hygiene

Fred F. Summerfelt

Abstract The 2010 Patient Protection and Affordable Care Act (PPACA) calls for midlevel dental healthcare providers to work in underserved areas with underserved populations. In 2004, Arizona passed legislation allowing qualified dental hygienists to enter into an affiliated practice relationship with a dentist to provide oral healthcare services for underserved populations without general or direct supervision in public health settings. The Northern Arizona University (NAU) Dental Hygiene Department has developed a teledentistry-assisted affiliated practice dental hygiene model that places a dental hygienist in the role of the midlevel practitioner as part of a digitally-linked oral healthcare team. Utilizing current technologies, affiliated practice dental hygienists can digitally acquire and transmit diagnostic data to a distant dentist for triage, diagnosis, and patient referral in addition to providing preventive services permitted within the dental hygiene scope of practice.

Keywords Patient Protection and Affordable Care Act • Training Materials • HIPPA • Training Methodologies • DICOM

5.1 Teledentistry-Assisted Affiliated Practice Dental Hygiene: A Workforce Model

In 2004, the Arizona Legislature approved a statute allowing qualified dental hygienists to enter into an affiliated practice relationship with a dentist to provide oral healthcare services for underserved populations without direct or general supervision in public health settings [5]. The United States Patient Protection and Affordable Care Act (PPACA), signed into law in March of 2010, greatly expands oral healthcare to eligible individuals [3]. To meet this increased need, midlevel dental healthcare providers will be needed to work with underserved populations in areas of professional isolation, which is an ideal opportunity for teledentistry-assisted affiliated practice dental hygienists.

F.F. Summerfelt, RDH, MEd
Department of Dental Hygiene, Northern Arizona University, Flagstaff, AZ, USA
e-mail: fred.summerfelt@nau.edu

S. Kumar (ed.), *Teledentistry*, Health Informatics,
DOI 10.1007/978-3-319-08973-7_5

5.1.1 *Affiliated Practice Dental Hygiene*

In 2004, the Arizona Legislature passed § 32–1289 that allowed qualified dental hygienists to enter into an affiliated practice to provide dental hygiene services without direct or general supervision pursuant to a written agreement, written procedures, and standing orders established by an affiliated dentist [5, 1]. In 2009, Arizona SB 1400 amended § 32–1289's limited patient demographic to include a person of any age who is either (a) enrolled in a federal, state, county, or local healthcare program; (b) participating in the national school meal program; (c) from a family with a household income of less than 200 % of the federal poverty guidelines; or (d) residing in a federally designated health professional shortage area. SB 1400 added additional language to § 32–1289 requiring patients treated by an affiliated practice dental hygienist to be examined by a licensed dentist within 12 months of initial treatment and that an affiliated practice dental hygienist must consult with the affiliated practice dentist before providing service to a patient with a complex medical history or medication regimen [4].

Arizona's affiliated practice dental hygienists are required to follow the standard of care for dental hygiene services. Specific qualifications for the affiliated practice dental hygienist include (a) a minimum of 5 years of dental hygiene experience; (b) active engagement in dental hygiene practice for at least 2,000 h in the 5 years immediately preceding the affiliated practice agreement; and (c) 12 additional hours of continuing education within the current triennial licensure renewal period, which must include 4 h of medical emergencies and a minimum of 8 h chosen from pediatric, special healthcare needs, preventive dentistry, public health, or community based dentistry [5]. See Table 5.1 for the procedures Arizona affiliated practice dental hygienists are allowed to perform.

5.1.2 *The Patient Protection and Affordable Care Act*

The 2010 PPACA calls for mandatory pediatric dentistry for eligible children up to age 21 and expands Medicaid to all who are at or below 133 % of the Federal Poverty Level [3]. Prior to the 2010 PPACA, the Surgeon General's 2001 report on oral health found vastly disproportionate availability of oral healthcare amongst certain American populations [6]. Since 2001, the increasing elderly population, the rising number of ethnic minority and immigrant populations, and the professional healthcare isolation present in many rural communities have added to the burden of providing oral healthcare for our diverse and already under-treated population. Additional considerations affecting future oral healthcare availability include the facts that, currently, two dentists will retire for each graduating dental student and enrolling dentists as Medicaid and PPACA providers will become more difficult due to burdensome administrative requirements [2]. The PPACA cites as examples of alternate dental workforce models Alaska's Dental Health Aide Therapist, the American Dental

Table 5.1 Procedures allowed for Arizona affiliated practice dental hygienists

Patient assessment	Preventive services	Patient education
1. Assess blood pressure	1. Perform all procedures necessary for a complete prophylaxis	1. Discuss patient's homecare procedures
2. Screen and photograph the oral cavity and surrounding structures	2. Apply dental sealants to teeth according to ADA and Centers for Disease Control and Prevention guidelines	2. Provide appropriate homecare instruction
3. Perform dental restorative charting and recording of clinical findings	3. Administer topical fluoride gels and varnishes as indicated according to ADA and Centers for Disease Control and Prevention guidelines	3. Provide tobacco cessation intervention and referral when appropriate
4. Expose and process dental radiographs according to ADA guidelines		
5. Perform a caries risk assessment		
6. Review medical and dental history		

Association's Community Dental Health Coordinator, and the American Dental Hygienists' Association's Advanced Dental Hygiene Practitioner [3].

5.1.3 NAU's Teledentistry-Assisted Affiliated Dental Hygienist Model

As an additional workforce alternative, NAU has pioneered an innovative teledentistry-assisted affiliated practice dental hygiene model to answer the call of the PPACA to provide comprehensive preventive oral healthcare and diagnostic services for the growing population of underserved in both urban and remote areas. Using current teledentistry technologies, dental hygienists can digitally acquire and transmit diagnostic data to a distant dentist for triage, diagnosis, and patient referral while providing all of the preventive services within their scope of licensure as part of a digitally-linked member of a oral healthcare team. NAU's digital diagnostic data acquisition equipment is state of the art and emerging technologies will only further the ability of distant dentists receiving the diagnostic data to properly diagnose, triage, and refer patients for appropriate treatment.

NAU's initial training endeavors prove that teaching the data acquisition technologies to dental hygiene students and dental hygienists has been easily and successfully accomplished. With only 6-h of training, dental hygiene students and dental hygienists have shown their ability to set up and manage remote patient-service facilities. While providing preventive oral healthcare services within the scope of affiliated practice, the dental hygiene students and dental hygienists have also acquired and forwarded digital diagnostically efficacious data from remote locations both using store-and-forward and cloud technologies

NAU's teledentistry-assisted affiliated practice dental hygiene has proven to serve the patient, the teledentistry-assisted affiliated practice dental hygienist, and the affiliated practice dentist. Patients benefit by the fact that they can receive preventive services locally, have their overall oral health evaluated by several members of a digitally-linked oral healthcare team, and schedule appropriate treatment with a minimum of travel and the associated costs of travel dollars and time off from work or out of school. Teledentistry-assisted affiliated practice dental hygienists benefit by being allowed to perform preventive services they are licensed to provide in a midlevel-practitioner model that promotes additional employment choices and professional opportunities. Affiliated practice dentists benefit by adding patients to their practice and filling their appointment schedules with patients receiving professional services only they can provide. The teledentistry-assisted affiliated practice dental hygiene model is easy to implement with existing technologies, provides a growing population of underserved with much-needed oral health services, and benefits all the members of the digitally-linked oral healthcare team.

5.2 Teledentistry Equipment and Training

In 2009, to develop the teledentistry-assisted affiliated practice dental hygiene workforce model and add teledentistry skills to its curriculum, NAU acquired two each of the following equipment:

1. Office management software
2. Digital imaging management software
3. Intraoral Digital Cameras
4. Digital x-ray film scanners
5. Portable hand-held X-ray units
6. Laptop computers
7. Projectors

All of the equipment chosen integrates seamlessly and has proven to be successful in both local and remote store-and-forward and cloud-based applications of teledentistry-assisted affiliated practice dental hygiene.

5.3 Teledentistry Training Materials

The NAU teledentistry curriculum has evolved over a 5-year period and has proven to be a successful hands-on educational program for interested parties, individuals intending to use teledentistry, and as a train-the-trainer apparatus for potential teledentistry educators. NAU has developed two specific tracks for teledentistry training including all required materials, visual presentations, participant handouts, and a teacher's manual to guide the visual presentations and classroom discussions. The first track is specific to informational presentations for interested community organizations, professional providers, and funders. The four informational courses include:

1. Teledentistry-assisted Enhanced Dental Teams
2. The Affiliated Practice Dental Hygienist
3. Teledentistry
4. HIPPA and Teledentistry

The second track, which requires 6–8 h of classroom time, is specific to dental professionals interested in learning about teledentistry, acquiring the hands-on skills and experience necessary to utilize teledentistry as part of a teledentistry-assisted enhanced dental team, and acquiring the knowledge necessary to become a teledentistry trainer. The seven courses, appropriate for both skill training and continuing education courses, include:

1. The Affiliated Practice Dental Hygienist
2. Teledentistry
3. HIPPA and Teledentistry
4. Training with Portable Hand-held X-ray Units
5. Teledentistry Equipment Set Up
6. Hands-On Training
7. The Future of Teledentistry

5.4 NAU's Training Methodologies

The professional-track teledentistry training methods and materials developed by NAU assume the students to be trained are either dental hygiene students or dental professionals trained in asepsis, radiography, and patient management. Training begins with familiarization of the various components of teledentistry equipment including the laptop computer, the software management system, the intraoral camera, a hand-held x-ray unit, a digital x-ray scanning device, phosphor plate x-ray films, a projector to project images for ease of operator use and as an educational tool for both patients and patient caregivers, and the various supplies needed to manage a remote nontraditional dental facility. Training should take place in an area large enough to have tables for the teledentistry equipment, a wall or screen to project images from the laptop computer, and a chair for an x-ray mannequin. The x-ray mannequin can be used by students to practice taking x-rays with the hand-held x-ray unit and become competent with the intraoral camera. Students can also acquire intraoral photographs from other students. An additional laptop or desktop computer and projector are required for student viewing of the various training modules. The seven professional track training modules are presented in order.

When training with the portable hand-held x-ray units, the manufacturer's training materials, narrated visual presentation, and competency test are used to assure all aspects of safety, unit management, and unit maintenance are thoroughly covered.

After students have learned to safely manage the portable hand-held x-ray unit, they are taught how to use the digital x-ray scanning device and manage the phosphor plate x-ray films. The digital x-ray scanning device scans phosphor plate x-ray films one or two at once. As the phosphor plate x-ray films pass through the digital x-ray scanning device, they are first scanned to the computer software program then exposed to a bright light, which erases the x-ray image from the phosphor plate. The operator must assure the digital x-ray scanning device erasure function is turned on to assure films are not double exposed.

Phosphor plate digital x-ray films come in all typical dental x-ray sizes and the digital x-ray scanning device has interchangeable ports specific to the size of the phosphor plate x-ray film chosen by the operator. Using the correct size port for the specific phosphor plate x-ray film size assures the plate passes through the scanner straight for optimal processing and viewing. The phosphor plate x-ray films are individually placed into sealable barrier packets with the font side of the plate facing the clear plastic side of the barrier. The solid black plastic side of the phosphor plate x-ray film barrier is positioned towards the source of the x-ray emission. The phosphor plate x-ray films have the letter "a" in the lower right corner of the film and this letter "a" is considered to be the raised dot on traditional x-ray films. When acquiring occlusal x-rays, NAU students are taught to use styrofoam bite blocks for occlusal x-rays to assure the patient does not bite down hard and damage the phosphor plate x-ray film. NAU students are taught the letter "a" is always placed into the slot of the styrofoam bite block used for periapical x-rays so the letter "a" does not occlude any of the patient's periapical area. Bite wing tabs are affixed to the black plastic side of the film barrier and placed in the patient's mouth as with traditional film bitewing x-rays. NAU students are taught to always place the letter "a" in the mandibular area of the bitewing x-ray to expedite the digital mounting process.

After exposing the x-ray, the phosphor plate x-ray films are ready to be processed. If only one operator is obtaining the x-ray series, the correct number of the correct size films should be barriered, exposed, and kept in a plastic cup within their barriers to prevent image degradation prior to the scanning process. When using this single operator method, the operator is able to keep his or her gloves on for the entire procedure and then open the film barriers in an aseptic manner upon completion of the x-ray image acquisition. The gloved single operator should open all of the exposed x-ray film barriers at once letting each film fall aseptically either blue side down on a counter top or directly into a black box to prevent the ambient light from degrading the x-ray image. Once all of the barriers are opened and the films aseptically removed, the single operator can remove her or his gloves and process all of the films in an expedient manner. If there are two operators, the gloved operator placing and exposing the phosphor plate x-ray films can open the barriers and allow the ungloved operator operating the digital x-ray scanning device to aseptically take the phosphor plate x-ray film from the opened barrier and immediately scan the film into the computer. Once the films have passed through the digital x-ray scanning device and been erased, they are ready to be barriered again for reuse. NAU students have conducted tests of phosphor plate x-ray film image degradation in ambient light and determined that a few minutes of exposure to ambient light once the phosphor plate x-ray film is removed from the film barrier does not degrade the digital image. Students learning to use the digital x-ray scanning device should be aware that they have a period of time that they can safely manage the exposed phosphor plate x-ray films in ambient light but should minimize the time as much as circumstances allow.

Management of the teledentistry-specific computer software during the time students are learning to acquire and scan digital x-rays should be managed by the trainer. Once the students have mastered the techniques of acquiring and scanning the x-rays, they should be taught how to manage the teledentistry-specific computer software. Assuming the students have basic knowledge of computer technology, the instructor should focus on utilizing the office image management software. Once in office management software program, the students are guided through the various functions of the software program including entering a new patient, locating a specific patient, acquiring patient-specific digital data from the digital x-ray scanning device, saving images, mounting images, and exporting images. Students should be familiarized with DICOM® and the need to export data electronically via the DICOM® module – store and forward data need not be exported via DICOM®. Students should be allowed to manipulate the software, import x-rays to a specific patient's record, and spend time managing individual x-ray images utilizing the various x-ray film manipulation functions within the office management software.

When students are competent with importing and managing x-ray imagery, they should move on to image acquisition utilizing the digital intraoral camera. NAU recommends utilizing a portable projector to project the intraoral image onto a wall or screen for ease of viewing and for patient and caregiver purposes. It is also advisable to select the full-screen mode in the image management software options. Students are first taught how to correctly barrier the intraoral camera to avoid a blurred image. The barriered intraoral camera prevents the need of a mouth mirror, a light, and sterilization equipment during teledentistry screenings. Students then gain experience positioning the intraoral camera with the x-ray mannequin. Buttons on the intraoral camera allow the operator to freeze the image for patient viewing and to acquire a photograph, which is immediately stored in the patient's chart. NAU students are taught to hold the intraoral camera against teeth of the opposite arch for maximum viewing area and steadiness while obtaining the photograph. Students are then shown how to aseptically remove the intraoral camera barrier. Once a new barrier is placed on the intraoral camera, students then obtain intraoral imagery from each other.

When students are competent in obtaining both digital x-rays and intraoral photographs, they are taught to mount and export the images. Office management software allows images to be entered into typical dental x-ray mounts via click-and-drag methodology. Mounts for bitewings, periapical, 18-shot fmx, and 20-shot fmx series are typically included. Custom mounts, which can contain intra- and extraoral photographs, are easily created. After mounting the films, students then learn to export the images. Typically, students are trained to export to store-and-forward devices such as thumb drives or CDs. Students are also shown how to export via DICOM® technology, which requires that the DICOM® module within the office management software to be turned on.

Once all the equipment-specific training is complete, the students are trained in assembling and disassembling the equipment. NAU has created a visual classroom presentation that shows, with a narrative, the step-by-step assembly methodology. Disassembling the equipment is not shown in the visual presentation but is inherently intuitive. Emphasis is always placed on the importance of secure packing of the equipment to prevent damage during transport. Students should be allowed to assemble, utilize the equipment to assure proper setup, and disassemble the equipment twice to assure competency. Additionally, students should use the printed handout from the visual presentation a guide to assembly in remote areas.

5.5 Teledentistry-Assisted Affiliated Practice Applications

The Northern Arizona Council of Governments (NACOG) Head Start program provides annual services to more than 1,500 preschool age children at 26 local centers in four counties covering 27,000 square miles of rural northern Arizona. Eighteen of the service centers are located more than a 3-h one-way drive from Flagstaff, where NAU is located. In 2009, NACOG Head Start contracted with a Flagstaff pedodontist to provide services for the Head Start children residing in the northern Arizona area. The NACOG-contracted pedodontist was aware of NAU's teledentistry-assisted affiliated practice model and saw the potential for teledentistry-assisted affiliated practice dental hygiene services to serve the Head Start population. Discussions between NAU, the NACOG Head Start manager, and the NACOG-contracted pedodontist led to an affiliated practice dental hygiene agreement, a pilot Head Start community outreach program, and a teledentistry-assisted affiliated practice demonstration model.

For the initial NACOG project, the teledentistry equipment was taken to United Way of Northern Arizona KinderCamps conducted at Flagstaff elementary schools. KinderCamp children include Head Start and preschool children from the Flagstaff Unified School District. Medical history and permission-to-treat forms had been signed by the KinderCamp children's primary caregivers prior to the events. On standing orders from the pedodontist, data including medical records, the chief complaint, head-and-neck examinations, existing conditions, intraoral photographs, and radiographs including occlusal views and bitewings were acquired. Fluoride varnish was applied to each child's teeth.

The public health screening atmosphere of the KinderCamp Head Start project proved the intraoral camera to be a very valuable asset. Placing a new barrier sheath over the camera before use with each child negated the need to use a mouth mirror and light for the assessment examination and provided a much better image of the intraoral area than could have been attained by a visual exam. A projector was used to enlarge the intraoral images onto a wall, which made it easy for the affiliated practice dental hygienist to see the intraoral images and the children enjoyed participating with their examinations because they could also see their teeth. The children liked the hand-held x-ray device and the use of the styrofoam bite blocks prevented accidental biting damage to the phosphor x-ray film plates used for occlusal views.

Following the 2 days of KinderCamp Head Start Screenings, the diagnostic data were forwarded to the NACOG-contracted pedodontist via a thumb drive. The pedodontist reviewed the diagnostic data and developed appropriate treatment plans for all of the children. The primary caregivers of the children were contacted directly by the pedodontist's staff to schedule appropriate treatment. The pedodontist found the pilot project to be successful and now uses teledentistry-assisted affiliated practice dental hygiene services in his practice.

Between October 2009 and the end of June 2010, the NAU participated with the Coconino County Maternal and Child Health Program to provide oral screening and appropriate teledentistry-assisted affiliated practice dental hygiene services for children participating in First Things First healthcare events at 13 different Coconino County locations. These activities took place within Flagstaff and at several remote Arizona sites including Williams, Page, Fredonia, Kaibab, Grand Canyon, and Supai. All of the remote areas were accessible by vehicle except Supai, which required the teledentistry team and equipment to be flown in by helicopter.

At each event, the team utilized the teledentistry equipment as the circumstances of the event allowed. Because of the lack of sterilization equipment and the need to move patients quickly through the process, the intraoral cameras with disposable sheath barriers proved very valuable in expediting the services. Projecting the intraoral images on the wall again proved to be advantageous because the dental hygienist could easily see large images of the intraoral environment and knew when to photograph areas of concern to be viewed later by the dentist.

One of the remote events, the Kaibab Health Fair, highlighted specific advantages offered by the teledentistry-assisted affiliated practice dental hygiene model for remote populations. Kaibab is 231 miles northwest of Flagstaff. The Paiute Indians living in the Kaibab area typically obtain dental services at the Hopi Health Care Center located in Polacca, which is 225 miles east of Kaibab. The NAU teledentistry-assisted affiliated practice team saw 23 children, including five children who appeared to need immediate care. The digital diagnostic data from the five children were forwarded to the Flagstaff-based affiliated dentist, who diagnosed the need for immediate care. The diagnostic data were then forwarded to the pedodontist at the Hopi Health Care Center. After reviewing the data, she instructed the NAU teledentistry coordinator to have the five children schedule immediate restorative services with her, thus eliminating the need for the children to first travel to Polacca, a 450-mile round trip, for an initial examination and treatment plan. The time and cost savings represented by the ability of the dentist to diagnose, triage, and treatment plan from digitally acquired data for these five patients exemplifies one of the teledentistry-provided advantages for remote populations.

5.6 Current and Future Applications of Teledentistry-Assisted Affiliated Practice

The success of the NAU teledentistry-assisted affiliated practice model has been well accepted by a growing number of Arizona community health organizations and oral healthcare providers. NAU is currently managing several teledentistry-assisted affiliated practice dental hygiene projects and establishing new relationships with dentists who can provide services for patients from Arizona's remotely located patient base. In addition to ongoing community demonstration projects, NAU is providing consultation, informative presentations, and hands-on training for community health organization personnel, dentists, and dental hygienists interested in establishing teledentistry-assisted affiliated practices in both Arizona and other states.

References

1. Goddard T. Attorney General opinion No. I05-009 (Ro5-013), A. R. S. § 32–1289 State of Arizona, 28 Dec 2005.
2. McKinnon M, Luke G, Bresch J, Moss M, Valachovic R. Emerging allied dental workforce models: considerations for academic dental institutions. J Dent Educ. 2007;71(11):1476–91.
3. Patient Protection and Affordable Care Act, U.S.C. H. R. 3950, 2010.
4. Senate Bill 1400 Amending Section 32–189, A. R. S. § 32–1289, 2009.
5. Title 32 Professions and Occupations, A. R. S. § 32–1289, 2004.
6. U.S. Department of Health and Human Services. Oral health in America: a report of the surgeon general. Rockville: U.S. Department of Health and Human Services, National Institute of Dental and Craniofacial Research, National Institutes of Health; 2000.

Chapter 6
Teledentisry and Dental Hygiene

Tracye A. Moore

Abstract The use of Teledentistry is the future of the way traditional dental practices will practice. Its use is controversial due to the cost of equipment, time for training of personnel, and lack of reimbursement for services billed. However, the many advantages range from reduced fees for patients to the increase use of dental hygienists, midlevel providers, and/or advanced dental therapists in non-traditional settings. Moreover, the use of Teledentistry affords underserved populations in rural and urban areas equity with regard to access to dental and medical services. For the facilitation of Teledentistry to be successful, the conversion of paper patient charts must be converted to a digital format (EHR or electronic health record) for radiographs, medical/dental histories, and prescriptions. The new millennium ushers the use of more computer systems, email, text messages, smartphones, and digital media for both the medical and dental professions in the inter-disciplinary approach to treatment of patients nationwide.

Keywords Electronic Health Records • SNODENT • Alaska Dental Health Aide Therapist • RDHAP

6.1 Introduction

Telehealth refers to the use of technology to provide health care at a distance [1]. Teledentistry and telemedicine are terms used to describe the use of dental and medical technology to facilitate interaction among patients and health care providers in geographically separated locations. These two terms have been combined and referred to collectively as "telehealth" [1]. The federal government has recognized that delivery of health care using telehealth technologies is a cost effective alternative to the more traditional face-to-face way of providing medical care [1]. Telehealth seeks to improve a patient's health by permitting two-way, real time interactive communication between the patient and the physician or practitioner at a distant site [1]. In order for telehealth to be successful, hospitals, dental offices, and medical

T.A. Moore, RDH, MS, EdD
Dental Hygiene Department, Northern Arizona University, Flagstaff, AZ, USA
e-mail: tracye.moore@nau.edu

S. Kumar (ed.), *Teledentistry*, Health Informatics,
DOI 10.1007/978-3-319-08973-7_6

offices should convert traditional paper patient records to multifunctional electronic health records (EHRs). The electronic health record should include both medical and dental information about a patient.

6.2 Electronic Health Records (EHRs)

To be considered multifunctional, EHRs need to have at least two of the following: a list of all patients' medications, a list of patients due for preventive care, electronic prescribing capabilities, and medical alerts about potential drug interactions [2]. The pace of EHR adoption in the United States has been accelerating since the passage of the Health Information Technology (HITECH) Act in 2009 which has made money available until 2021 to encourage hospitals, doctors, and other caregivers to adopt EHRs [2]. In 2009, President Obama signed into law the American Recovery and Reinvestment Act, which has aided in the expansion of broadband and wireless service and mandated that by 2015, all medical records, including dental, must be converted to an EHR [3]. Barriers to adoption of electronic health records include: financial (start-up costs of hardware and software and the uncertainty of payment for services); technical (lack of computer skills or lack of technological training); time (to convert paper records to electronic and to learn the system); psychological (people resist change); social (fear of lack of communication with patients); privacy (security and HIPAA concerns); and organizational (practitioners in larger practices may be more receptive to EHR adoption than those in smaller practices) [1, 2]. Dentists and dental hygienists should be prepared for the nationwide adoption of EHRs.

6.3 EHRs and SNODENT

For the dental profession, there is no fixed deadline to switch to EHRs; however, for those dentists who bill Medicare for patient services, starting in 2015, Medicare reimbursement rates will be affected if the meaningful use (using the EHR to electronically send prescriptions to pharmacies) of EHRs has not been demonstrated [4]. For traditional billing, there will be no impact on reimbursement; however, for the dentists who bill Medicare, there will be reductions in Medicare payments to providers who do not adopt EHRs by the end of 2014 [4]. In preparation for the fast approaching deadline, in 2007 the American Dental Association (ADA) created a task force which worked towards creating an individual online database system called Systemized Nomenclature of Dentistry (SNODENT®) [3, 5]. SNODENT® is an internationally recognized system of vocabulary and codes designed to use in the electronic environment for electronic health and dental records globally. Its purpose is to: provide standardized terms for describing dental disease; capture clinical dental and patient characteristics; permit analysis of patient care services and outcomes;

and to be interoperable with EHRs [5]. The benefits of using SNODENT® include: improved communication among dentists and other health care providers; improved patient care through evidenced-based practices; enhanced data collection to evaluate oral care outcomes; enhancement of public health investigation and reporting; and greater capability to measure adherence to standards of care [5]. The use of SNODENT® by dental professionals as the standard for electronic dental records will prepare them for patients who cross state lines seeking dental treatment.

6.4 The Implementation of National EHRs

When patients need medical and/or dental treatment in another state other than the one in which they are domiciled, how is medical information transferred when paper records are destroyed? Are the dental and medical professions prepared for a natural disaster that could affect the medical and dental records of millions of Americans? In 2005 after Hurricane Katrina, one of the most deadliest hurricanes ever to hit the United States, several states partnered in an effort to help make sure their residents' health information is available after a hurricane or wide-spread disaster. Working with the Department of Health and Human Services Office of the National Coordinator for Health IT (ONC), health information exchange (HIE) programs in Alabama, Georgia, Louisiana, Florida, South Carolina, North Carolina, Virginia, Michigan, Wisconsin, and West Virginia partnered in 2013 which will allow for HIE among providers caring for patients who are displaced from their homes [6]. After disasters like Hurricanes Katrina, Sandy, and Oklahoma, patients benefit more when states and HIE organizations work together to ensure that health information can be readily accessed when patients need it the most. The Southeast Regional Health IT and Health Information Exchange Collaboration (SEARCH) established in 2010, which members include Alabama, Arkansas, Louisiana, Georgia, Mississippi, North Carolina, South Carolina, Kentucky, Tennessee, and Virginia have collaborated, using a variety of methods, to help resolve cross-border barriers toward facilitating the multi-state exchange of health information [6]. This health information includes both electronic medical and dental records of patients displaced by natural disasters.

6.5 Types of Dental EHRs

There are several different type of EHR software programs dental schools, offices, and organizations can use such as Dentrix®, PracticeWorks®, EagleSoft®, and MOGO™ to allow for more efficient communication and reduction of a paper trail among providers, specialists, and telehealth sites in rural areas [3]. All of these different software applications allow for: electronic dental claims management; sending electronic prescriptions; incorporation of patients' medical history, dental

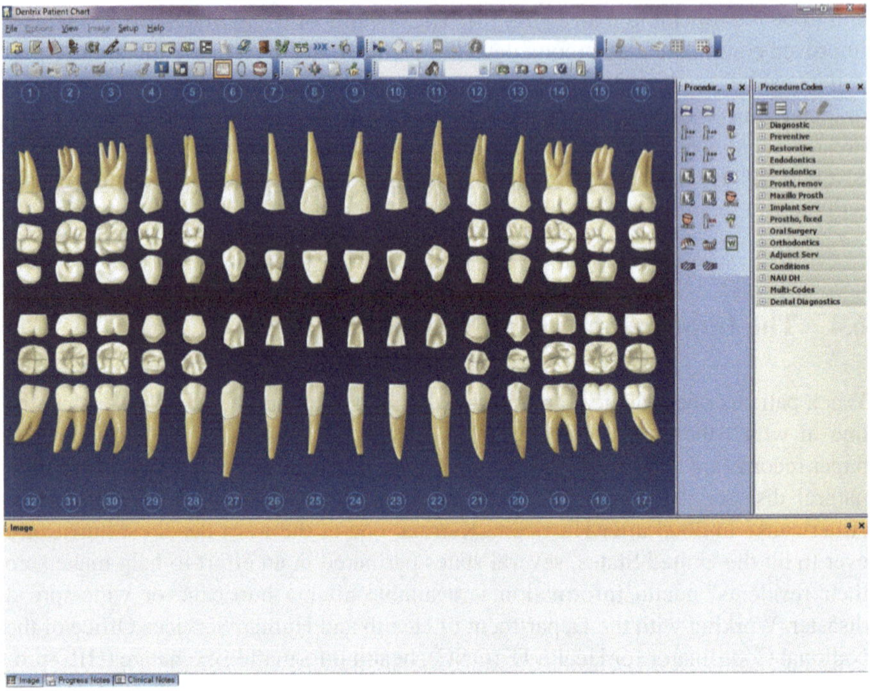

Fig. 6.1 Patient electronic dental record. Dentrix screenshot courtesy of Henry Schein Practice Solutions, American Fork, Utah (Reprinted with permission)

radiographs, periodontal charting, and dental charting (see Fig. 6.1); the ability for patients to complete their registration and medical histories online; taking patients pictures with a webcam; record findings verbally; importing and exporting images into the patients' files; using digital signatures or fingerprint technology to identify users; backing-up patient records virtually, and more recently, using a smart phone, mobile device, or tablet to access current patient information [7–10]. There are various companies that provide the aforementioned software programs and choosing the software which is right for your type of practice should be determined by: user-friendly ability for practitioners (and patients based on literacy levels); cost for software installation, staff education, and tech support; customization capabilities for dental documents; and EHR security and confidentiality. Although the use of dental EHRs has just begun to gain prominence, its use dates back to the early 1900s.

6.6 The History of Teledentistry

Telemedicine began in 1924, with the concept of a physician seeing his patient over the radio using a television screen [11]. The initial concept of teledentistry developed as part of the blueprint for dental informatics, which was drafted at a 1989 conference funded by the Westinghouse Electronics Systems Group in Baltimore

[12]. The birthplace of teledentistry as a subspecialist field of telemedicine can be linked to a 1994 military project of the United States Army Total Dental Access Project aiming to improve patient care, dental education, and effectuation of the communication between dentists and dental laboratories [3, 11–13]. Teledentistry was put into practice by the U.S. Army by doing consultations on persons located more than 100 miles apart [11]. Since that time, various public health facilities, remote rural clinics, and organizations have practiced teledentistry with various degrees of success. The variation in the levels of acceptance and use of dental EHRs throughout the profession has been determined by the mode of communication preferred, type of software and hardware used, and the type of internet connection.

6.7 Methods of Communication

Teleconsultation through telehealth can take place either in "real-time" or "store-and-forward" methods [3, 11–13]. Real-time consultation involves a videoconference (see Fig. 6.2a) in which dental professionals and their patients, at different locations, may see hear, and communicate with one another actually using advanced telecommunication technology and ultra-high bandwidth network communications [11–13]. Store-and-forward (see Fig. 6.2b) refers to the collection and secure transmission of encoded information including patient documents and images (intraoral photos, radiographs, and extraoral photos) which are stored for review by a dentist or specialist at a later time for consultation and treatment planning [3, 11–13]. A third method has also been described, known as "remote monitoring method" in which patients are monitored at a distance and can either be hospitalized or home-based [12]. Since the patient is not present during the store-and-forward consultation, dentists can share patient information, radiographs, photos, and other information transportable through multiple providers [12]. This data sharing can be of extreme importance for patients in need of a specialist who may not be located nearby, patients who have been displaced by natural disasters who need treatment, and patients who may need to be monitored at a distance.

6.8 Technological Requirements

To practice dentistry within the realm of telehealth, a desktop or laptop computer with a microphone and substantial hard drive memory are needed. In addition, a significant amount of RAM with a speedy processor; a digital camera, video camera and intraoral camera for the capture of pictures [11, 12]; and a portable x-ray unit (NOMAD®) (see Fig. 6.3) are essential. A comprehensive software capable of image acquisition and storage, and transmission of the gathered information and software capable of coding and decoding audio and video is desirable [11]. A fax machine, scanner, and a printer may also be required in some cases [12]. There is great variation in levels of speeds to connectivity to the internet and broadband technology, increasingly widespread and available, offers a selection of cutting-edge

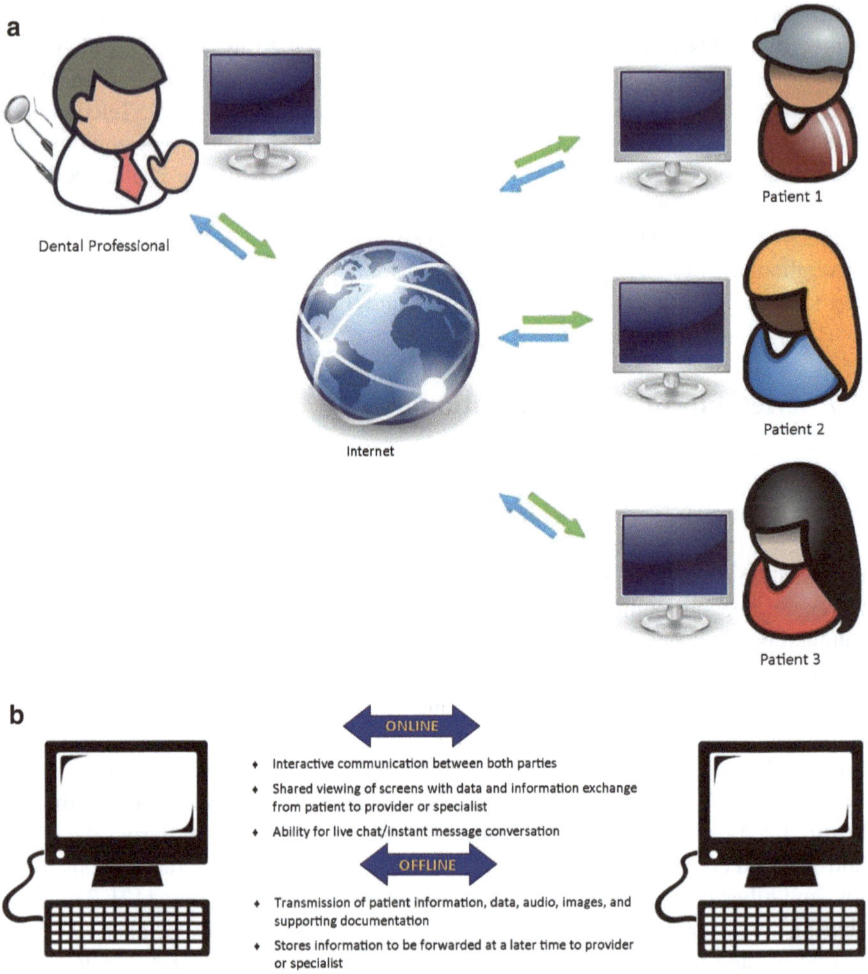

Fig. 6.2 (**a**) Type of teleconsultation. (**b**) Types of telecommunication

alternatives well suited to meet the needs of the telehealth professional and his or her staff [11]. There are many advantages as well as disadvantages to using telehealth technology.

6.9 Advantages of Using Teledentistry

Teledentistry provides a unique way to help overcome the barriers or geography and travel time to deliver long-distance clinical training, continuing education, and hands-on training for the dentist/dental hygienist at remote clinics [11, 15].

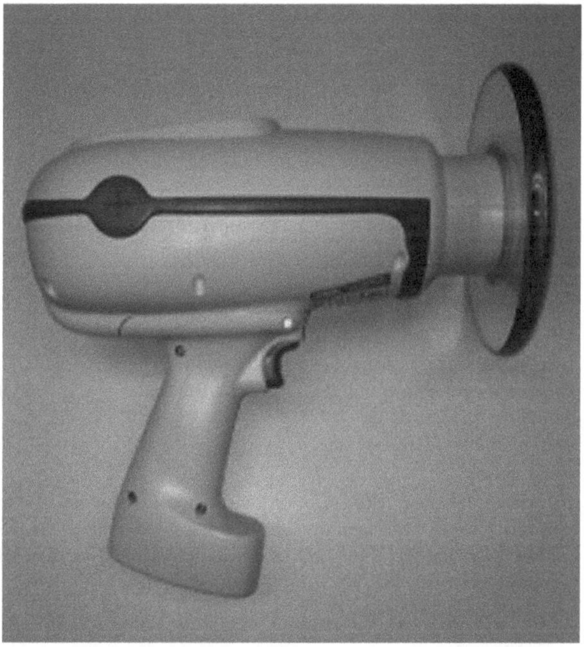

Fig. 6.3 NOMAD® handheld portable radiograph unit (Photo of actual equipment)

Its application is of utmost importance and great value in rural and urban underserved areas where there is unavailability of specialist consultation which reduces the costs of service and improves quality of care [12–14]. The results of telehealth usage increase inter-professional communications which will improve dentistry's integration into the larger health care delivery system [13]. Second opinions, pre-authorizations and other insurance requirements will be met almost instantaneously online, with the use of real images of dental problems, thereby making traditional dental care more efficient [14, 15]. In addition, it will facilitate the greater use of nondentist providers (such as dental hygienists or mid-level providers) and improve early diagnosis and treatment of oral disease [15]. For dental and dental hygiene schools, interactive video-conferencing allows for the evaluation of patient information (with or without the patient's presence), which allows for the interaction and feedback between the educator and the students [14]. Telehealth can serve as a tool to compliment and expand the capacity of school child care centers to meet the children's dental care needs by using technology to connect to the health providers at another location [14]. For dental facilities, there is long term cost effectiveness due to savings generated from not purchasing equipment and materials to develop traditional dental radiographs. Although Telehealth is being used nationally and internationally by educational institutions and public health facilities, still many legal, financial, and ethical concerns exist (Table 6.1).

Table 6.1 Teledentistry advantages

Financial	Social	Technical
Increased use of dental hygienists, advanced dental therapists, and mid-level providers	Delivery of dental services to remote areas	Second opinions, pre-authorizations, and insurance requirements met via electronic dental claims management
Increased interaction of educators and students at dental and dental hygiene schools via video-conferencing	Treatment of underserved rural or urban populations	Early diagnosis of dental problems via email, the use of smartphones, tablets, or mobile device to access patient records
Increased capacity of school child care centers meeting the dental needs of children thereby reducing emergency room visits	Increased inter-professional communications	Virtual back-up of electronic medical and dental health records can be used across state lines to facilitate more efficient patient treatment
Increased revenue due to non-purchase of materials for traditional radiograph development	May provide equality in the provision of dental and medical healthcare services	Convenient patient access to complete medical and dental histories online

6.10 Disadvantages of Using Teledentistry

Telehealth allows the dental hygienist to initiate treatment based upon their assessment of a patient's need without a dentist on site; however, supervision levels vary from state to state and this affects the services a dental hygienist may perform in rural and remote settings using teledentisty equipment [3]. Accountability, licensure, jurisdiction, liability, privacy, consents, and malpractice are crucial aspects to consider when attempting to establish the foundations of a telehealth practice [11, 13]. The most significant barrier to a nationwide teledentistry practice is the traditional system of state-by-state licensing. There is no law to clarify the role of the teledoctor and their liability [11]. The cost of the telecommunication equipment has also been a matter of concern and presently, the cost for virtual teledental consultations has not been reimbursed by insurance companies [3, 12]. Ethically, patients must be made aware that their medical and dental information will be transmitted electronically and the possibility exists that the information will be intercepted, despite maximum efforts to maintain security and confidentiality [11, 13]. In addition, some doctors may use the internet to set up and seek direct patient contact, thus becoming cyberdentists [11, 13] using telehealth technology. Other challenges include: the time and cost it takes for practitioners and staff to get acclimated to using the telehealth system. In underserved communities (below the poverty line) located in rural or urban areas, the lack of infrastructure and patient literacy remain major obstacles (Table 6.2).

Table 6.2 Teledentistry disadvantages

Financial	Social	Technical
Liability and malpractice for dental hygienists and dentists	Supervision rules of dental hygienists vary from state to state	Privacy of electronic health records may be compromised
Cost of telehealth software and hardware equipment	Accountability of practitioner	Virtual patient consent
Cost to train personnel to use equipment	Dentists may abuse virtual diagnosis capability	Training time of dentist and staff to learn how to use equipment
Uncertainty of payment for services	State by state licensure and jurisdiction	Lack of infrastructure to accommodate high speed internet lines

6.11 Teledentistry Use by Dental/Dental Hygiene

There are several states that have been at the forefront of the use of telehealth technology: Alaska, Minnesota, and California. According to Dr. Mary Williard, Director of the Alaska Dental Health Aide Therapist (DHAT) Training Program, "Since the 1990s, Alaska has been an international leader in telehealth technology. The DHATs and most all healthcare providers in Alaska's Tribal Health System use telehealth technology provided by the Alaska Federal Health Care Access Network (AFHCAN). AFHCAN is a for profit company run by the Alaska Native Tribal Health Consortium. All of our village clinics have their telehealth carts. We also use telephones and email. Many providers access children in the villages by going to the schools. These services would be enhanced by the use of laptop computers through which electronic health records can be accessed" (M.E. Williard, DDS, email communication, August, 2013).

Apple Tree Dental in Minnesota is a nonprofit dental practice that operates five regional dental access programs in urban and rural areas of Minnesota [1]. Tele health technologies link special care dental clinics with on-site dental clinics at schools, Head Start Centers, group homes, assisted- living centers, nursing facilities, and other community sites for people facing physical, financial, and geographical barriers [1]. The Apple Tree model links dental hygienists working under "collaborative agreements" with dentists [1]. Approximately 70 % of children in Head Start Centers being served need only preventive services provided by the dental hygienist [1]. For the 30 % who need treatment by a dentist, this is provided by a dentist who comes on site with portable equipment [1].

The Pacific Center for Special Care at the University of the Pacific, Arthur A. Dugoni School of Dentistry located in San Francisco, California created a "Virtual Dental Home" complete with a collapsible dental chair, laptop computer, digital camera, supplies to do temporary fillings, an internet-based dental record system, and a handheld x-ray machine where registered dental hygienists in alternative practice (RDHAP), registered dental hygienists working in public health programs (RDH), and registered dental assistants (RDA) provide care to underserved populations in schools, nursing homes, community centers, and Head Start centers [16–19]. These teams led by geographically distant dentists can keep many people healthy in community settings by providing triage, case management, preventive procedures, and early intervention therapeutic services [16]. Telehealth technology allows for the medical histories and dental images to be uploaded to a website where a dentist reviews them and creates a treatment plan or refers patients requiring more complex treatment to a dentist in the area [19]. Telehealth has the potential to provide underserved patients with oral healthcare services in addition to being a beneficial tool to decrease the disparity and ensure equality in provision of oral healthcare services [20].

6.12 Summary

Currently, the use of teledentistry has not yet become an integral aspect of oral health care; however, its implementation is necessary for the sustainment of our society. It is imperative that medical and dental providers support the use of telehealth by dental hygienists and mid-level providers in non-traditional settings where access to care for underserved communities is a challenge. Dental and dental hygiene schools will benefit from the use of telehealth technology because interdisciplinary and inter-professional learning for college students will become enhanced. The use of telehealth technology will help bridge the geographical divide between the community provider and the dentist. Medical and dental students will become educated and trained through virtual service-learning projects which may encourage many (after graduation) to invest their skills in underserved rural or urban communities.

The mandate of EHRs combined with the technology to facilitate dental care at remote sites has set the stage for the execution of telehealth clinics all over the United States and internationally. However, several issues must be addressed before telehealth will become widespread such as: the various laws and jurisprudence regarding dental and dental hygiene licensure and the financial and geographical barriers faced by rural populations. The future of telehealth is dependent upon federal grants to continue the development of telehealth programs in dental and dental hygiene schools, public health facilities, and other organizations; the use of reimbursable codes by dental professional for the use of technology and virtual visits; and the national promotion of the use of dental hygienists and mid-level providers in non-traditional settings.

References

1. Glassman P, Helgeson M, Kattlove J. Using telehealth technologies to improve oral health for vulnerable and underserved populations. J Can Dent Assoc. 2012;40(7):579–85.
2. Porter M. Adoption of electronic health records in the United States. Kaiser Permanente Executive Summary. 2013;1–7. http://xnet.kp.org/kpinternational/docs/Adoption%20of%20Electronic%20Health%20Records%20in%20the%20United%20States.pdf. Accessed 15 July 2013.

3. Williams KT. The use of teledentistry to provide dental hygiene care to rural populations. Access. 2011:1–6. http://www.thefreelibrary.com/The+use+of+teledentistry+to+provide+dental+hygiene+care+to+rural...-a0275853707. Accessed 15 July 2013.
4. Electronic health records frequently asked questions. American Dental Association website. https://www.ada.org/sections/dentalPracticeHub/members/ehr_faqs.pdf. Published 2011. Updated 2013. Accessed 15 July 2013.
5. Systemized nomenclature of dentistry (SNODENT). American Dental Association website. http://www.ada.org/snodent.aspx. Updated 2013. Accessed 15 July 2013.
6. States prepare for seamless exchange of health records. Health and Human Services website. http://www.hhs.gov/news/press/2013pres/07/20130711a.html. Published 11 July 2013. Updated 5 Aug 2013. Accessed 15 July 2013.
7. Dentrix practice management software features. HenrySchein/Dentrix website. http://www.dentrix.com/products/dentrix/digital-dental-office/. Updated 2012. Accessed 15 July 2013.
8. CS PracticeWorks software features. Carestream Dental/CS PracticeWorks website. http://www.carestreamdental.com/us/en/practicemanagement/PRACTICEWORKS#FeaturesandBenefits. Updated 2013. Accessed 15 July 2013.
9. Eaglesoft software benefits and features. Patterson/Eaglesoft website. http://patterson.eaglesoft.net/PracticeManagementCharting/Overview. Updated 2013. Accessed 15 July 2013.
10. Mogo dental software features. Mogo website. http://www.mogo.com/operatory.shtml. Updated 2013. Accessed 15 July 2013.
11. Sanjeev M, Shushant GK. Teledentistry: a new trend in oral health. Int J Clin Cases Investig. 2011;2(6):49–53.
12. Jampani ND, Nutalapati R, Dontula BSK, Boyapati R. Applications of teledentistry: a literature review and update. J Int Soc Prev Community Dent. 2011;1(2):37–44.
13. Bhambal A, Saxena S, Balsaraf SV. Teledentistry: potentials unexplored. J Int Oral Health. 2010;2(3):1–6.
14. Chhabra N, Chhabra A, Jain R, Kaur H, Bansal S. Role of teledentistry in dental education: need of the era. J Clin Diagn Res. 2011;5(7):1486–8.
15. Skillman SM, Doescher MP, Mouradian WE, Brunson DK. The challenge to delivering oral health services in rural America. J Public Health Dent. 2010;70:S49–57.
16. Glassman P, Harrington M, Namakian M, Subar P. The virtual dental home: bringing oral health to vulnerable and underserved populations. J Can Dent Assoc. 2012;40(7):569–76.
17. Lauer G. Telehealth project brings virtual dental home to patients. California Healthline. 2013. http://www.californiahealthline.org/insight/2013/telehealth-project-brings-virtual-dental-home-to-patients. Accessed 21 Aug 2013.
18. University of the Pacific. Dental school pilots telehealth project in San Mateo County. Pacific Insider. 2013. http://www.pacific.edu/About-Pacific/Newsroom/2013/May---August-2013/Dental-School-Pilots-Telehealth-Project-in-San-Mateo-County.html. Accessed 21 Aug 2013.
19. Graeber L. Virtual dental homes care for vulnerable populations. California Health Report. 2013. http://www.healthycal.org/archives/10842. Accessed 21 Aug 2013.
20. Khan SA, Omar H. Teledentistry in practice: literature review. Telemed J E Health. 2013;19(7):565–7.

Chapter 7
Access to Oral Care Through Teledentistry

Susan J. Daniel and Sajeesh Kumar

Abstract It has been reported that in the US, there are 4,230 geographic areas that experience dental care shortage, many of which are rural or remote areas without dental professionals. Some researchers have suggested that teledentistry might be a solution to this problem, especially in effective screening for dental caries in young children. Teledentistry is the use of information technology and telecommunications for dental care, consultation, education, and public awareness; teledentistry is similar to other types of telehealth. Dental hygienists can perform clinical screenings for carious lesions, yet in some states, dental hygienists are not permitted to do so by law. Once a patient has been screened by a dentist, the dentist may authorize the dental hygienist to perform specific functions under "general supervision," meaning that the dental hygienist can perform only those functions authorized.

Keywords Access to Care • Teledentistry • Dental Hygiene • Oral Care

It has been reported that in the US, there are 4,230 geographic areas that experience dental care shortage, many of which are rural or remote areas without dental professionals [1]. Some researchers have suggested that teledentistry might be a solution to this problem, especially in effective screening for dental caries in young children [2, 3]. Teledentistry is the use of information technology and telecommunications for dental care, consultation, education, and public awareness; teledentistry is similar to other types of telehealth [4]. Dental hygienists can perform clinical screenings for carious lesions, yet in some states, dental hygienists are not permitted to do so by law. Once a patient has been screened by a dentist, the dentist may authorize the

S.J. Daniel, RDH, PhD
Chairman and Associate Professor, G.W. Hirschfeld School of Dental Hygiene,
2011 College of Health Sciences, Old Dominion University, Norfolk, Virginia 23529, USA

S. Kumar, PhD
Department of Health Informatics and Information Management,
University of Tennessee Health Science Center, 920 Madison Avenue Suite 518,
Memphis, TN, 38163, USA
e-mail: skumar10@uthsc.edu

S. Kumar (ed.), *Teledentistry*, Health Informatics,
DOI 10.1007/978-3-319-08973-7_7

dental hygienist to perform specific functions under "general supervision," meaning that the dental hygienist can perform only those functions authorized.

Teledentistry screening can provide early referral for care before patients develop quality of life issues and loss of teeth due to dental caries. The aim of this study is to identify whether a difference in early screening for dental caries exists between dental hygienists and dentists using either clinical or teledentistry methods.

7.1 Epidemiology of Dental Caries

In 2000, the Surgeon General of the United States called dental caries a "silent epidemic" and the "single most common chronic childhood disease" [5]. Data from the 1988–1994 NHANES-III revealed that more than half of 5-year-old children who are living below the poverty line and children whose families' earnings barely meet daily needs but do not qualify for federal assistance had dental caries that was essentially untreated [6]. As an infectious disease left untreated, dental caries can have serious effects on other body systems that can eventually result in sepsis and death [7–11]. Data from more recent surveys (e.g., data from 1999–2004 NHANES) have furthered supported the increased prevalence of dental caries in preschool children with low socioeconomic status [12].

To combat the silent epidemic of dental caries, the Surgeon General recommends "screening and early detection to arrest the progress of the disease after it occurs" [5]. Two measures associated with dental caries screening are prevalence and extent. Prevalence is defined as any carious lesion that is severe enough to result in cavities and necessitates restoration [6]. Prevalence is often reported using the index for decayed and filled teeth; whereas, extent of dental caries is measured by an index for decayed and filled surfaces (DFS) [6].

The index for DFS is used to identify the number of surfaces on each tooth that are affected by decay. To obtain a DFS score, each tooth is divided into five surfaces, and each surface filled with decay is tallied as one point. For example, if one tooth had four surfaces with decay and another tooth had one surface with decay, the DFS score would equal 5. DFS scores differ from decayed and filled primary teeth (DFT) scores because DFS scores are based on the total amount of decay but DFT scores are based on the number of teeth having any decay. For example, if a child has 20 teeth but only two present with carious lesions, the DFT score would be 2. The DFS score for the same child with the two teeth identified with decay would require a total of the involved surfaces.

Data from 1988–1994 NHANES-III indicated that 2-year-olds with low SES averaged one-half DFT, and 5-year-olds had greater than 2.7 DFT [6]. The same data set also revealed that 2-year-olds with caries had more than three cavities per child regardless of SES [6]. However, SES was not found to affect caries prevalence among children 3–5 years of age: Severity of dental caries was the same for children from low SES and near low SES households. Even though SES did not seem to affect caries prevalence among 3- to 5-year-olds, half of the 5-year-olds with low or near low SES who had dental caries were untreated [6]. More recent data

Table 7.1 Dental caries experience and untreated caries by age for children 3–5 and 6–9 years

	Dental caries experience filled or unfilled		Untreated dental decay	
	Age 3–5 (%)	Age 6–9 (%)	Age 3–5 (%)	Age 6–9 (%)
Gender	33.3	54.4	23.8	28.8
Male	35.4	56.8	24.5	30.1
Female	31.2	51.7	23.1	27.4
Ethnicity				
Hispanic/latino	47.2	70.3	34.5	41.4
Non-hispanic/latino	–	–	–	–
Caucasian	29.2	50.0	20.1	25.1
African American	36.8	55.6	27.5	35.7
Origin of birth				
Inside US	32.7	53.9	23.2	28.2
Outside US	49.7	63.3	40.2	41.1
Insurance status				
Insured	31.8	53.9	22.2	27.4
Private	25.2	46.7	17.7	21.8
Public	43.5	69.6	30.1	39.7
Uninsured	45.4	59.7	38.0	37.9

Note. Adapted from two sources: (1) "Dental caries experience: children 3–5 years (percent)," by Health Indicators Warehouse, n.d. Retrieved from http://healthindicators.gov/Indicators/Dental-caries-experience-children-3-5-years-percent_1269/Profile/Data; (2) "Dental caries experience: children 6–9 years (percent)," by Health Indicators Warehouse, n.d. Retrieved from http://health-indicators.gov/Indicators/Dental-caries-experience-children-6-9-years-percent_1270/Profile/Data

(1999–2004) from the ongoing NHANES indicated 23.8 % of children age 3–5 years and 28.8 % of children aged 6–9 years had untreated dental caries [12]. Thirty-three percent (33.3 %) of 3- to 5-year-olds and 54.4 % of 6- to 9-year-olds had either filled or unfilled dental caries. (Table 7.1) In short, the literature supports evidence of increased prevalence of dental caries in children 2–5 years of age and decreased prevalence in older children. Literature also indicates that regardless of age, dental caries is largely untreated [6].

Pain from dental caries in children has been reported by parents and caregivers in several studies. Reports of pain from dental caries in 3- to 5-year-old children are as high as 68.0 % in Canada [13], followed by 16.0 % in the UK and Maryland [14] and 14.9 % in North Carolina [15]. In a Maryland study, 8.9 % of Head Start children were reported to cry from pain associated with dental caries [14]. Additionally, results from these and other studies have also revealed that children who have dental caries suffer from difficulty eating and sleeping [13, 16].

Dental caries affects the quality of life for children. Children can often describe how they feel when asked. Caregivers were asked questions about their children's oral health and other items reflecting quality of life, and then, the children were asked to select either a happy face or sad face to describe their feelings about their teeth. Of the caregivers whose children had severe caries ($n = 77$), 27.0 % reported absenteeism from school, 31.0 % said their children were ashamed to smile, and 49.0 % reported their children had difficulty eating. Thirty-seven percent of children who had severe caries were more likely to select a sad face than were the 22.0 % of children who did not have severe caries [17].

7.2 Development of Dentition and Early Care

Most caregivers understand that the primary teeth will be lost and replaced by permanent teeth. Losing the first primary tooth is sign of growth and development and, therefore, receives much attention. When children begin to exfoliate primary anterior teeth, parents and children focus oral care not on the posterior portion of the mouth but on the eruption of the emerging permanent anterior teeth. At approximately the same time that the primary central incisors are being exfoliated and replaced by the permanent incisors, the first permanent molar emerges posterior to the last primary molar. It is easier to see visible decay on an anterior tooth than on a molar, so thorough oral hygiene and self-care are often neglected for newly erupted molars, which can result in oral environments that are conducive to dental caries. Therefore, early screening for childhood caries is critical to children's overall health and development.

Primary and permanent teeth have different anatomical features: The occlusal surface of primary molars has shallow pits and fissures, but the occlusal surface of permanent molars has deeper pits and fissures, allowing not only for better mastication of food but also for increased collection of plaque biofilm and food debris. If parents and children focus oral care primarily on newly emerging anterior teeth, newly erupting posterior teeth (e.g. molars) may not be cleaned as well as needed, thus creating oral environments that are conducive to development of dental caries.

7.3 Access to Care

In the US, there are 4,230 geographic areas that experience dental care shortages, many of which are rural or remote areas without dental professionals [1]. In 2009–2010, the number of individuals without health insurance in the US increased by over a million [18]. The resulting statistics indicate there are currently 108 million people in the US without dental insurance; furthermore, there are only approximately 141,800 working dentists and 174,100 working dental hygienists [18]. Because of the low numbers of working dentists and dental hygienists and the high number of individuals who need dental care, individuals in rural areas are less likely to have access to care due to location of health services and lack of health-care providers.

People living in both rural and urban areas can experience trouble accessing dental care. According to the U. S. 2010 census, 82.3 % of the US population lived in urban areas where dental health-care professionals prefer to live and work. Access to care in urban areas is not due to a deficit of oral care providers, but like people living in rural areas, those living in urban areas share some of the same concerns that often prevent people from seeking care and that contribute to disparities in care (e.g., lack of funds, insurance, transportation, education, knowledge, and beliefs that dictate oral health-seeking behaviors [19].

Health insurance does not always include dental coverage because traditionally, health insurance has meant medical coverage exclusive of dental coverage. In fact, more people have health or medical insurance than dental insurance [20]. People who have health insurance without dental coverage typically obtain dental coverage through a separate policy for only dental insurance.

In 2012, Congress passed the Patient Protection Affordable Care Act (PPACA) to fill coverage gaps left by traditional health insurance [21]. Because PPACA is still being developed and implemented, the extent of dental care coverage provided through PPACA is still unclear, although it does seem as if PPACA will help make dental coverage available for children [21]. Nevertheless, exactly who and what will be actually covered in the PPACA is still a concern, especially because of the $64 billion spent annually on dental care, only 4.0 % was paid by government programs [1].

In addition to geographical location and lack of dental coverage, access to dental care is further restricted by lack of uniform regulations in licensing dental professionals [22]. Licensure of dental professionals and the tasks assigned to each specific professional group of dental professionals are governed by each state. Individual states establish their own dental practice acts containing rules and regulations governing practices and functions of oral care professionals and levels of supervision required for non-dentists who provide care for patients, including dental hygienists.

There are a few states (e.g., Colorado and California) where dental hygienists can practice either independently from or collaboratively with dentists [23]. In these states, dental hygienists can screen for disease, diagnose, plan, and provide services without the permission or authorization of licensed dentists. Unlike dental hygienists, midlevel practitioners with specific licensure and expanded-functions certifications have more flexibility to practice oral care in Arizona and Minnesota [23–25]. For example, midlevel practitioners in Minnesota and Alaska not only provide preventive services but also perform restorative services and simple extractions. Many dental hygienists have the skills and knowledge to perform expanded functions and are licensed by their states and by the American Dental Association National Board for Dental, so practice restrictions for dental hygienists reduce the ability to meet the dental needs of the population and impede the access to oral care.

In summary, health-care disparities and barriers such as SES, geographical location, lack of insurance, and lack of uniform regulations inhibit reliable access to proper screening and treatment for dental caries. These barriers and disparities have lead dental health professions to look for new ways to connect with patients. Some researchers believe that these barriers to care can be overcome through the use of telehealth and teledentistry, which represent the next frontier of medicine [26].

7.4 Dental Caries Screening by Dental Hygienists

Clinical screening for dental caries can be performed by a dentist, by a dental hygienist, or by both depending on the dental practice laws of the state. The American Dental Hygienists' Association reported in 2013 that only 24 states currently allow dental hygienists to conduct clinical screenings for diseases in the oral cavity [22]. The remaining 26 states do not allow dental hygienists to conduct clinical screenings, but dental hygienists can use teledentistry for screening, diagnosis, and referral for treatment of dental caries without the physical presence of a licensed dentist. As such, teledentistry screening for dental caries is an auxiliary means of addressing access-to-care issues that should be furthered researched.

In each of the five studies in the literature that incorporated teledentistry for screening of dental caries, intraoral images were captured and transmitted for remote screening and were compared to clinical screening of the same participants [2, 3, 27–29]. In one of these studies, researchers compared intraoral images to clinical examination findings [27]. In another, a dental examiner calibrated the DSTM for quantifiable validity and reliability of dental caries assessment using visual examination (i.e., DFS > 0 if a lesion was present and DFS = 0 for no lesion) and screened a convenience sample of 50 children aged 4–6 years from an inner city preschool [30]. Images of the children's teeth were obtained following the examination. Two weeks later, the images were scored by the same dental examiner using the same DSTM scale. Reliability between the two screenings was reported as the following: $\kappa = .61$ with 100.0 % sensitivity and 81.0 % specificity [27]. This level of agreement and accuracy provides evidence that teledentistry screening is a valid and reliable method of screening for dental caries.

In another study, telehealth assistants obtained six intraoral images on 162 preschool children and then transmitted the images to a remote site where a dental examiner assessed caries prevalence. Results indicated that 43.0 % ($n = 69$) of the children had either early childhood caries (ECC) or severe early childhood caries (S-ECC). The mean DFS score was 1.88 ($SD = 3.49$), and the range of DFS scores was from 0–20 surfaces. ECC was noted in 48 of the 69 children with a DFS score of 4.42, and S-ECC was noted in 28 of the 69 children with a DFS score of 7.61. Of the 28 children diagnosed with S-ECC, 6 had a DFS score of ≥6 [28].

Four dentists were partnered in another study to remotely diagnose dental caries in 66 children aged 4–6 years using intraoral images obtained by trained childhood educators. The remote diagnoses were compared to the clinical diagnoses of an experienced dentist's clinical examination of the same children. The comparison yielded the following results about the two types of diagnoses: sensitivity of 94.0–100.0 %, $\kappa = 52.0$–100.0 %. Agreement among the pairs of dentist examiners ranged from moderate to high as indicated by the Kappa statistic, and the identification of teeth that were positive for dental caries was very high as indicated by the percentages of sensitivity. At the conclusion of the study, half of the children ($n = 33$) required referrals for further care [2].

Teledentistry provides a methodology for dentists and dental hygienists to obtain screening data, remotely diagnose dental caries, and authorize treatment without being physically present, thereby increasing access to care for children who have limited or no access to care [29].

7.5 Recent Findings

The authors recently completed a study comparing clinical and teledentistry screenings for dental caries, performed by dental hygienists and dentists using both methods. The study used a convenience sample of 82 children 4–7 years of age. Participants attended schools in Memphis, Tennessee, USA and were provided preventive and educational services by students enrolled at the University of Tennessee Health Science Center's Dental Hygiene Program. Memphis is located in Shelby County, which has a population of 927,644. Nearly 20.0 % (19.7 %) of the county population is in the poverty category. African Americans comprise over 51.9 % of the population in Shelby County [31]. Memphis charter schools are 97.6 % African American, and non-charter schools are 82.4 % African American.

Mobile equipment was brought into the schools and a licensed dentist examined children prior to the delivery of preventive care. A licensed dental hygienist supervised dental hygiene students during the provision of preventive services as required by the practice act in Tennessee. Participants had to be 4–7 years old with completed informed consent by their parents or guardians. Seventy-eight children met the inclusion criteria for the study. There were four examiners: a clinical dentist and dental hygienist and a teledentistry dentist and dental hygienist; each consented to participate in the study.

Each child received a clinical screening by the dentist for dental caries and existing restorations, and findings were recorded on a geometric chart. At a separate visit, the dental hygienist completed a clinical screening for caries and existing restorations recording clinical findings on a second dental chart.

Following the second clinical screening intraoral images were obtained on each child. The number of images per child varied based on the number required to obtain the desired anatomy. Dental anatomy captured on all children included the anterior teeth in occlusion and the occlusal surfaces of all molars. The Apple iPhone 4S® was used and found to provide the most efficient and effective means for obtaining images on children as this is a familiar device and not intimidating. The zoom feature was used to obtain anatomy in the posterior region. Cheek retractors and intraoral mirrors were used to obtain images of the anatomical features most associated with carious lesions in young children. Children were shown how to place the cheek retractors and were engaged in the process.

Photos were stored in digital albums by subject number, uploaded to the cloud and stored in a secure file for access only by the Principal Investigator and the teledentistry examiners. Each teledentistry examiner reviewed the photographs, and

Table 7.2 Frequencies and percentages for categorical demographic variables

	n	%
Gender		
Male	27	37.0
Female	46	63.0
Screening age		
4	13	16.7
5	19	24.4
6	14	17.9
7	32	41.0
Ethnicity		
African American	56	71.8
Caucasian	4	5.1
Hispanic	18	23.1
Grade in school		
Prekindergarten	17	21.8
Kindergarten	11	14.1
First grade	26	33.3
Second grade	24	30.8

Note. Frequencies not summing to $N=78$ reflect missing data

recorded existing restorations and dental caries on separate charts. Findings on each chart were given a DFS score and the four scores were compared.

Descriptive findings can be seen in Table 7.2. Sixty-three percent (63 %) were females, 72 % African Americans, 41 % 7 years of age and 64 % were from the first and second grades. Spearman's Correlation's compared with the clinical dentist (CD) and clinical dental hygienist was $r=.993$, followed by CD and teledentistry dental hygienist $r=.808$ and the CD and teledentistry dentist $r=.753$.

The Wilcoxon Sign Ranks test found no significant difference ($p>.10$) in DFS scores between the clinical dentist and the teledentistry dental hygienist.

The findings from this study suggest that a dental hygienist's clinical findings of dental caries are nearly the same as those of the clinical dentist based on the correlation coefficient. Of equal importance is that there was no statistical difference in the assessment of caries by a dental hygienist using teledentistry and the same assessment performed by a clinical dentist.

7.6 Implications for Access to Care

The current literature on use of teledentistry for assessment of dental caries and other oral conditions provides evidence that this methodology is advantageous in providing access to populations in need of care. Whether used as a screening mechanism or as a component pared with electronic radiographs and health record including chartings, teledentistry can provide all the required data at the minimum to make a referral and in many cases, a diagnosis of certain oral conditions and subsequent treatment.

Dental hygienists and expanded functions oral care providers who do not have the authority to diagnose and treat due to restrictive practice regulations could obtain the electronic data, store and forward to an offsite dentist for review, diagnosis and authority to treat the patient according to the needs presented within the realm of the care provider's professional license. Teledentistry would allow for delivery of oral care to rural and urban groups, individuals in long-term care, special needs populations and many others who do not have access to oral care.

Advocacy and policy change is needed to make the use of Teledentistry a universal reality. Additional evidence is needed in multiple populations and geographic regions to support change and access to care using teledentistry.

References

1. Public health, oral health statistics. http://www.hrsa.gov/publichealth/clinical/oralhealth/.
2. Amavel R, Cruz-Correia R, Frais-Bulhosa J. Remote diagnosis of children dental problems based on non-invasive photographs–a valid proceeding? Stud Health Technol Inform. 2009;150:458–62.
3. Kopycka-Kedzierawski DT, Billings RJ. Prevalence of dental caries and dental care utilization in preschool urban children enrolled in a comparative-effectiveness duty. Eur Arch Pediatr Dent. 2011;12(3):133–8.
4. Clark G. Teledentistry: what is it now, and what will it be tomorrow. J Calif Dent Assoc. 2000;28(2):121–7.
5. U. S. Department of Health and Human Services. Oral health in America: a report of the surgeon general. Rockville: National Institute of Dental and Craniofacial Research; 2000.
6. Tinanoff N, Kanellis M, Vargas C. Current understanding of epidemiology, mechanisms and prevention of dental caries in preschool children. Pediatr Dent. 2002;24:543–51.
7. Slavkin HC, Baum BJ. Relationship of dental and oral pathology to systemic illness. JAMA. 2000;284(10):1215–7.
8. Offenbacher S, Lin D, Strauss R, McKaig R, Irving J, Barros P, Moss K, Barrow D, Hefti A, Beck JD. Effects of periodontal therapy during pregnancy on periodontal status, biological parameters and pregnancy outcomes: a pilot study. J Periodontol. 2006;77(12):2011–24.
9. Albert DA, Begg MD, Andrews HF, Williams SZ, Ward A, Conicella ML, Rauh V, Thomson JL, Papananou PN. An examination of periodontal treatment, dental care, and pregnancy outcomes in an insured population in the United States. Am J Public Health. 2011;101(1):151–6.
10. Scannapiecco FA, Ho AW. Potential associations between chronic respiratory disease and periodontal disease: analysis of National Health and Nutrition Examination Survey III. J Periodontol. 2001;72(1):50–6.
11. Offenbacher S, Beck JD, Moss K, Mendoza L, Paquette DW, Barrow DA, Couper DJ, Stewart DD, Falkner KL, Graham SP, et al. Results from the Periodontitis and Vascular Events (PAVE) Study: a pilot multicentered, randomized, controlled trial to study effects of periodontal therapy in a secondary prevention model of cardiovascular disease. J Periodontol. 2009;80(2):190–201.
12. Dye BA, Tan S, Smith V. Trends in oral health status: United States, 1988–1994 and 1999–2004. In: Centers for Disease Control and Prevention, editor. Vital health stat. Washington, DC: Health and Human Services; 2007. p. 248.

13. Low W, Tan S, Schwartz S. The effect of severe caries on the quality of life in young children. Pediatr Dent. 1999;21:325–6.
14. Vargas CM, Monajemy N, Khurana P, et al. Oral health status of preschool children attending Head Start in Maryland. Pediatr Dent. 2000;24:257–63.
15. Pahel TB, Rozier RG, Slade G. Parental perceptions of a children's oral health: the Early Childhood Oral Health Impact Scale. Health Qual Life Outcomes. 2007;5:6–16.
16. Nuttall NM, Steele JG, Evans D, Chadwick B, Morris A, Hill K. The reported impact of oral condition on children in the United Kingdom. Br Dent J. 2003;200:551–5.
17. Feitosa S, Colares V, Pinkham J. The psychosocial effects of severe caries in 4-year children in Recife, Pernambuco, Brazil. Cad Saude Publica. 2005;21:1550–6.
18. Centers for Disease Control and Prevention. Vital signs: health insurance coverage and health care utilization – United States, 2006–2009 and January–March 2010. In: Morbidity and mortality weekly report, vol. 59. Rockville: Health and Human Services; 2010. p. 1–7 (Early Release).
19. Edelstein BA. Disparities in oral health access to care: findings of national surveys. Ambul Pediatr. 2002;2(Suppl):141–7.
20. Bloom B, Cohen RA. Dental insurance for persons under age 65 years with private health insurance: United States, 2008. NCHS Data Brief #40. Hyattsville, MD: National Center for Health Statistics, Centers for Disease Control and Prevention, U.S. Department of Health and Human Services, 2010. http://www.cdc.gov/nchs/data/databriefs/db40.htm.
21. Health insurance reform what does it mean for dental and vision plans. http://www.benefitmall.com/News-and-Events/Legislative-Updates/Health-Insurance-Reform-What-Does-It-Mean-for-Dental-and-Vision-Plans.
22. American Dental Hygienists' Association: Dental hygiene practice act overview: permitted functions and supervision levels by state. In: ADHA; 2012: chart. Chicago, Illinois.
23. Gurav A, Jadhav V. Periodontitis and risk of diabetes mellitus. J Diabetes. 2011;3(1):21–8.
24. Feidt A. Report calls for expansion of Alaska's dental health therapist model. Anchorage: APRN; 2012.
25. Nash DA. Envisioning an oral healthcare workforce for the future. Community Dent Oral Epidemiol. 2012;40(Suppl S2):141–7.
26. Doolittle GC, Williams AR, Cook DJ. An estimation of costs of a pediatric telemedicine practice in public schools. Med Care. 2003;41(1):100–9.
27. Kopycka-Kedzierawski DT, Billings RJ, McConnochie KM. Dental screening of preschool children using teledentistry: a feasibility study. Pediatr Dent. 2007;29(3):2099–213.
28. Kopycka-Kedzierawski DT, Bell CH, Billings RJ. Prevalence of dental caries in Early Head Start children as diagnosed using teledentistry. Pediatr Dent. 2008;30(4):329–33.
29. Patterson S, Botchway C. Dental screenings using telehealth technology: a pilot study. J Can Dent Assoc. 1998;64(11):806–10.
30. Fyffe HE, Deery C, Nugent ZJ, Nuttall NM, Pitts NB. In vitro validity of the Dundee Selectable Threshold Method for caries diagnosis (DSTM). Community Dent Oral Epidemiol. 2000;28(52–58):52.
31. Tennessee demographics, Shelby County. http://www.tennessee-demographics.com.

Chapter 8
Forensic Odontology in Digital Era

Kelly Tanner Williams and Brenda Tallon Bradshaw

Abstract A major purpose of forensic odontology is the medicolegal establishment of human identification. The focus is often for cases of unidentified human remains or for bitemark investigations of criminal activity. With advanced technologies, forensic odontology is able to efficiently accomplish these tasks with accuracy. The cost and limited accessibility of advanced equipment sometimes hinders widespread utilization. Still, a basic understanding of what exists and is available can support structured growth. This chapter will link modern technologies to the way odontologists collect, organize, interpret, and document evidence in their professional practice to offer a basic understanding of how teledentistry is being applied in forensic odontology.

Keywords Medicolegal • Forensic odontology • Postmortem • Antemortem • Global positioning system • Digital radiography • X-ray fluorescence spectrometer • RFID tag • 3D computerized reconstructions • Unified Victim Identification System • UVIS Dental Identification Module • Bitemark analysis • Root-transparency level • Daubert Guidelines

8.1 Background

A major role of forensic odontologists is that of assisting with human identifications for deceased individuals. Such cases could be within the context of identifying one victim in a local morgue or thousands of victims in a temporary morgue established for a mass fatality incident (MFI). Methods used to obtain positive medicolegal identifications are similar for both situations. The identification process includes postmortem (PM) evaluations, antemortem (AM) collection and interpretation, followed by a comparison phase of all evidence. The concept of using unique oral features to positively identify a person has very early roots. Possibly the earliest documented example took place in the

K.T. Williams, RDH, MSDH
Old Dominion University, Gene W. Hirschfeld School of Dental Hygiene,
16111 Rhodes Lane, Chesterfield, VA 23838, USA
e-mail: ktwillia@odu.edu

B.T. Bradshaw, RDH, BSDH
Old Dominion University, 1600 Holly Point Lane, Suffolk, VA 23436, USA
e-mail: bbrad006@odu.edu

S. Kumar (ed.), *Teledentistry*, Health Informatics,
DOI 10.1007/978-3-319-08973-7_8

first century BC when the Roman Empress Agrippina requested confirmation of an ordered assassination. The victim's head was delivered to the Empress so that the victim's misaligned dentition could serve as proof [31]. A 1776 silversmith dentist, Paul Revere, was able to identify the decomposing body of someone wearing an ivory and silver wired denture he fabricated [31]. While these historic cases relied heavily on visual memorization, present day cases are built on unrefutable scientific proof and aided by modern teledentistry technologies. Cases of murder, abuse, and MFIs such as the September 11, 2001 terrorist attacks, Hurricane Katrina, and the 2004 Asian tsunami have relied heavily on the expertise of forensic odontologists.

8.2 Human Remains Investigations

8.2.1 Digital Photography

For unknown deceased victims, collection of odontological evidence begins in the location where the human remains were found. Typically, collected human remains are given to the custody of a coroner or medical examiner working closely with a forensic odontologist by local authorities or disaster search and recovery authorities as opposed to the odontologist being onsite. However, depending on circumstances, the odontologist may need to report to the scene where the remains were discovered in order to obtain more odontological evidence [15, 31]. In such cases, photographic documentation of the site with global positioning system (GPS) coordinates as a part of that evidence can assist in relocating the exact site with certainty [37]. A high-quality 35 mm single-lens reflect (SLR) digital camera with adjustable exposure settings and changeable lenses is recommended for taking multiple photographs [32]. Extra- and intraoral photographs should be taken of the victim and used to compare PM information against AM information [14, 32]. Digital photographic images can be electronically stored, retrieved, and wirelessly transmitted for additional expert opinion.

8.2.2 Digital Dental Records and Radiography

Human remains identification by odontological means relies heavily on the comparison of AM and PM dental records. The AM data collections team works with the victim's dentist of record in order to obtain needed information [11]. While paper records are accepted and used, electronic records are preferred for several reasons. Paper records take longer to obtain, they are often illegible, film-based radiographs have to be digitized with a flat-bed scanner, and the record with its contents have to be monitored to avoid misplacement [10, 22]. In contrast, electronic dental records are wirelessly transmitted for quick retrieval and they are in easy to read type print with radiographs already in digital format.

PM digital radiography with portable radiation emitting, hand-held units is the preferred method for forensic odontology victim evaluations [23]. Since digital images can be magnified for image-spot scrutiny, they allow for quality requirements that are essential to forensic odontology; such as, clear cementoenamel junction outline, clear pulpal outline, detailed root apex contour, and restoration margin discriminations [23, 30]. Digital radiography is also logistically beneficial for a couple of reasons. First, using digital radiography conveniently eliminates the need for chemical developer solutions or darkrooms [31]. Additionally, the use of small portable, hand-held x-ray units eliminates the need for access to facilities with fixed wall units, making on-site use possible [23, 30]. Limiting the need for the body to be transported to another site prior to taking dental radiographs is of particular importance in situations of fragility when moving the body could result in physical damage, which would reduce the ability to continue gathering quality information due to deterioration [15]. Portable radiation emitting units include the AnyRay, Nomad, Rextar, and MinRay, and digital image receptors include the Durr PSP, Sigma M CMOS, Sopix, DEXIS, and VistaRay CCD [14, 23, 31]. Time saving direct digital image receptors with charged couple device (CCD) or complementary metal oxide semiconductor (CMOS) pixels can be wirelessly directed to a computer [14]. Digital radiography images can be viewed instantly, allow for exposure correction manipulations, and can be retaken as needed so that quality can be obtained [14]. Digital radiographs are also easily and readily uploaded into comparison software so that identification matches can be computed [14]. If additional expert opinion is desired, tele-radiology allows digital radiographs to be viewed from a distant site when used in universal imaging format, digital imaging and communications in medicine (DICOM) [31] Fig. 8.1.

With increasing use of dental cosmetic resin restorations, it is sometimes difficult to visually and radiographically scrutinize modern restorations in order to make needed comparisons [31]. Laboratory based scanning electron microscopy with energy dispersive X-ray spectroscopy (SEM/EDS) used in conjunction with the spectral library identification and classification explorer (SLICE) software can help identify resin material in an extracted tooth (Bush et al. 2008). Another resin identification method option used in the morgue or field is the portable X-ray fluorescence

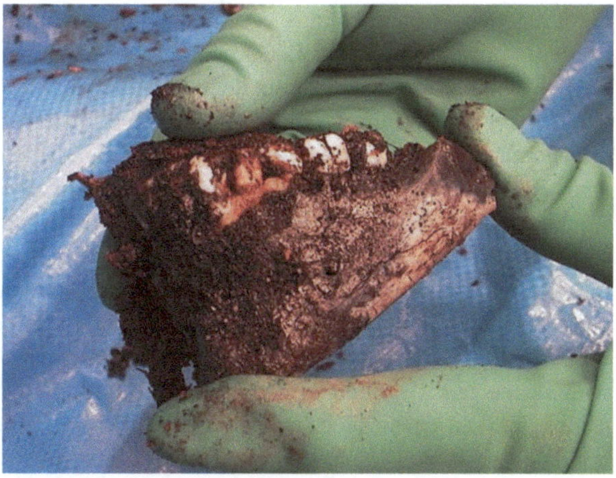

Fig. 8.1 This is a burn victim identification case where the lower jaw was removed to facilitate the taking of radiographs. The anterior teeth are completely charred, however the remaining sockets can be useful in identification

spectrometer (XRF) paired with a custom spectral library database to identify manufactured brands of resin dental materials ([4, 5]; Bush et al. 2008). Dentists should have the victim's AM record noted with the brand names of restorative materials used so that information gathered by the SEM/EDS or XRF can help add to the certainty of identification ([4]; Senn and Stimson 2010). Still, AM and PM dental radiographic comparisons are the main odontological method used for identifications, but when traditional methods have been exhausted, SEM/EDS and XRF may be needed [4].

8.2.3 Cone-Beam Computed Tomography

Three-dimensional imaging in the form of cone-beam computed tomography (CBCT) is gaining popularity for clinical diagnostics and treatment planning in dental specialties. These highly detailed images become a permanent part of the patient's dental record, and could serve as sources of AM information. Forensic odontologists can also use CBCT in order to obtain PM information, especially in cases when intraoral access and 2 dimensional (2D) dental radiography are not possible [14].

8.2.4 Computed Tomography, Magnetic Resonance Imaging and Surface Scanning

Enough detailed information from the deceased victim needs to be obtained in order to compare against AM data so that a positive identification can be confirmed. However, this is sometimes to achieve due to physical manipulation difficulty or religious objections to invasive means raised by the victim's family [19]. In cases where PM dental information needs to be obtained, but is not possible through invasive surgical means, computed tomography (CT) is an option [19, 29]. This advanced three-dimensional (3D) digital radiography system yields detailed information while leaving the body intact. When available, mobile CT scanner vehicles equipped with distance reporting telecommunications could assist efforts at a MFI temporary morgue or onsite for crash accidents [29]. Comparisons of 2D dental radiographs are considered the gold standard for establishing dental unique identifiers, but CT images can be utilized as a complementary tool [3]. While sometimes criticized for its inability to give discriminatory information that is detailed enough for comparing dental restorations, it has been found to be valuable for age estimation in cases involving child victims [3].

When CT is combined with magnetic resonance imaging (MRI) and surface scanners, a non-invasive virtual autopsy makes it possible to obtain a large amount of PM information; including dental [11, 18]. An example of such a system is the Virtopsy project, which relies on a robotic system guided by three-dimensional surface scanning and software in order to collect autopsy information on fragile human remains without the risk of physical damage to the body [9, 28]. To begin, a digital SLR camera and optical surface scanner collect photogrammetry and triangulation imagery data that is wirelessly communicated to a software responsible for calculating millions of surface points on the skin, which navigate a robotic arm on how to perform the virtual autopsy task [28]. If the equipment is available during DVI events occurring in remote areas, the planning and commanding of the robotic arm can be carried out through wireless communications by experts who are off-site [9]. Virtual autopsy is a new and very advanced technique which is still being studied [19].

8.2.5 *Radio Frequency Identification Tags*

Using dental records to identify a person by unique characteristics found within the dentition is a common and well rehearsed activity among odontologists [26, 27]. However, identifying an edentulous person can be quite challenging due to the loss of unique odontological identifiers; making marked dentures invaluable for edentulous victims [20]. Methods for labeling oral prostheses ranges from surface notations in the form of handmade engravings or pen marks, to structural inclusion techniques such as thin papers, film or metal labels with a clear protective coating [8, 26]. These methods tend to be cost effective, simple to accomplish, and make identification easier than having no markings at all. However, they can have drawbacks in the form of esthetics, the potential for trapping bacterial plaque, and being susceptible to not holding up to the destructive nature of extreme heat, acids, or wear [8, 26]. Alternative methods that are quick and easy to access include electronic information storing microchips, barcodes, or radio frequency identification tags (RFID tag) that can be structurally included into the denture [7]. A major benefit of RFID tag use is its durability against harsh assaults such as extreme heat, freezing temperatures, wear, or acid exposures [26]. The wireless electronic communication data carrying tag contains a microchip with an antenna and is rated to have an unlimited lifespan [26, 27]. Identification information is accessed by a mobile handheld reader with an electromagnetic field emitting antenna to energize the transponder (tag). The tag gives the coded data to the reader, which translates the data into readable information [25]. Information stored on the tag can be changed over time as needed and is capable of holding contact information in addition to the name of the wearer.

8.2.6 *Three-Dimensional Craniofacial Reconstruction*

Forensic odontological and anthropological examinations of skeletonized remains can offer evidence of age, gender, and ethnicity so that a 3D craniofacial reconstruction can recreate an AM likeness [33, 34]. This is particularly important when there is no source of AM information for the unknown victim [6]. Advantages of 3D computerized reconstructions over traditional manual clay methods includes time efficiency, less subjective influences, characteristic variations can be applied for multiple renderings, and the digital image can be easily shared from a distance [17]. When the resulting image is released to the public, someone may recognize the victim and come forward to give authorities information to aid the investigation [6].

8.2.7 *Software and Databases*

Identifying a deceased victim relies heavily on comparisons of collected AM and PM dental information. Comparison software such as WinID3, Plass Data's DVI System, and Unified Victim Identification System (UVIS) enables collected data to be electronically catalogued and filtered [14, 37]. Software algorithms automate comparisons based on dental patterns and other unique identifiers so that records can be ranked by numbers of matches, mismatches, and possible matches [2]. Prior to such software systems, odontologists spent a lot of time manually comparing multiples of AM records against each PM record of interest that was within their possession [14]. In addition to saving a lot of time, these software systems can be compared against databases for missing persons since they have a high probability of being a deceased victim odontologists will attempt to identify. Missing persons databases available for searches in multiple languages include UVIS Dental Identification Module (UVIS/UDIM) and NamUS (the National Missing and Unidentified Persons System) [36, 37]. These databases are accessible by the internet and can assist in the identification of unknown human remains [36, 37].

8.3 Bitemark Investigations

8.3.1 *Bitemark Identification*

Bitemarks are prevalent in cases where a victim has attempted to defend themselves from a perpetrator. A bite can be defined as a mark made by human or animal teeth on the skin of "living individuals, cadavers, or objects with relatively softened consistence" [13], p. 45. Bitemark analysis can be of assistance to the forensic team when attempting to understand if time has elapsed between the production of the mark and the examination. Analysis can also assist to determine if the marks occurred antemortem or postmortem, and in the case of multiple bites, the sequence of bite production can yield useful information [13] Fig. 8.2.

Bitemarks can be located anywhere on the body, however they are most often identified in areas of soft, fleshy tissues such as the face, stomach and buttocks [18]. When identifying bitemarks on a victim and dental records are not available, unusual oral characteristics gleaned from the teeth are used to narrow down clues based on the biter's lifestyle habits such as wear patterns, chipping of teeth, dietary patterns, and socioeconomic strata [18]. In addition to unique conditions present, identifiers such as formation of eruption and dental aging based on cementum-formation and root -transparency level may assist in analysis of the data.

A bitemark is the result of a mandibular closure, followed by negative pressure (suction), in the opposite direction, "caused by the tongue and peri-oral musculature" [13], p. 46. When a person or animal bites an object, the upper incisors hold the object while the lower incisors cut. The marks that are left are relevant to inform

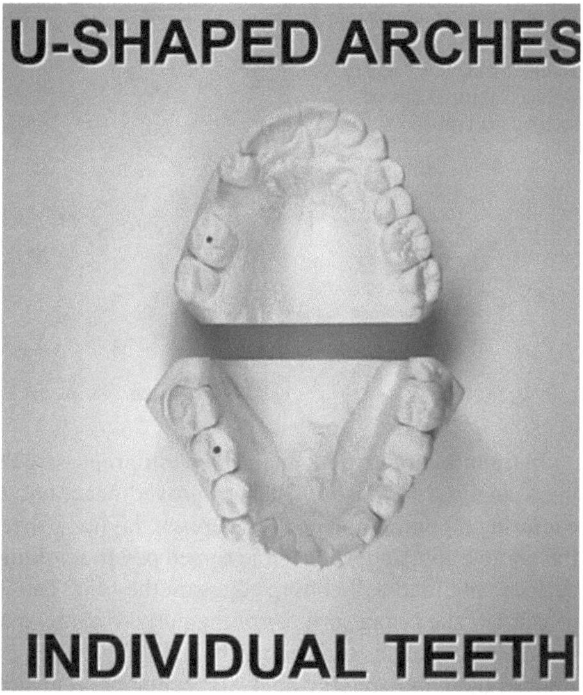

Fig. 8.2 Indicates the criteria for recognizing a bitemark as human

the bitemark analysis on details such as "dental alignments, size, and shape of dental arches" [13], p. 46. Human dentition is unique to each individual because each of the teeth in the dentition has its own size, shape, and features. Additionally, factors such as past dental extractions, restorations, malalignment, malformation, interdental spacing, and dental fractures can also be detected in the analysis. Bitemark analysis is very difficult on human skin because of distortion that may be present or time elapsed between the production and analysis. Other factors such as applied force, bite duration, and movement between the skin and the teeth also may affect the lesions produced during the incident [13].

8.3.2 *Bitemark Analysis Techniques*

Advanced technologies have been made available within the manufacturing industry that are more accurate traditional overlay methods. A three-dimensional analysis of bitemarks are made possible by using a calibrated digital camera to capture images of the bitemark. Advances within the technology of the calibrated camera accommodate for scale and angulation distortion of the bite. The scanned image is then able to produce a model of the teeth that accurately represents a dentition that closely replicates that of the offender. A disadvantage of utilizing the advanced technology is the initial cost of the equipment. In the case where advanced technology is cost-prohibitive, traditional methods of bitemark analysis are also very reliable Fig. 8.3.

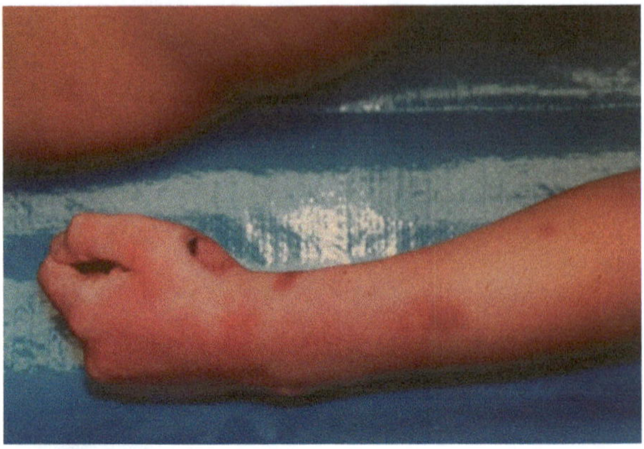

Fig. 8.3 A bitemark on the left hand of a homicide victim. Numerous "defensive wounds" (bruises can be seen on her arm)

In traditional bitemark analysis, photographs are the primary method for bitemark analysis because of their improved accuracy. Bitemark analysis involves capturing a photograph of the bitemark, laying a sheet of transparency film over the photograph, and using a fine tipped pen to marking the perimeter of the biting surface, and marks the biting edges on the film. The film is then used as a means to validate the biting surfaces of the perpetrator by matching it to the drawing. In the manual analysis technique, the actual teeth are compared to the transparent film. In the photocopying analysis technique, a positive reproduction of the perpetrator's teeth have been fabricated (i.e. dental models) and has been laid incisal edge down on a photocopier to produce a photocopied image. The image is then placed upside down on a radiographic view box where the teeth were outlined on the transparency film, and the outlines are compared. In computer assisted methods, the dental models of the perpetrator are scanned with the biting edges of the dental models over the glass plate of a scanner and are then transferred to a computer or laptop. The images are opened utilizing Photoshop 7 ™, and the biting edges are reproduced and printed on a transparent sheet of paper. A comparative study of overlay methods was conducted by Khatri et al. [16] and their study concluded that the most consistent and reliable means of comparing the three overlay analysis was that of the computer assisted overlay generation Figs. 8.4 and 8.5.

8.3.3 Accidental and Nonaccidental Injuries

Accidental and nonaccidental injuries exhibit distinctly different characteristics. Nonaccidental, or abusive clinical signs are that of fractured teeth, cuts, fractured nasal and jaw bones. Additionally, such markings as cigarette or ligature burns or such as bitemarks on the face, neck, or arms are signs of clinical abuse [18]. In child abuse cases, there are characteristics of abusive injuries that are prevalent with the case. One

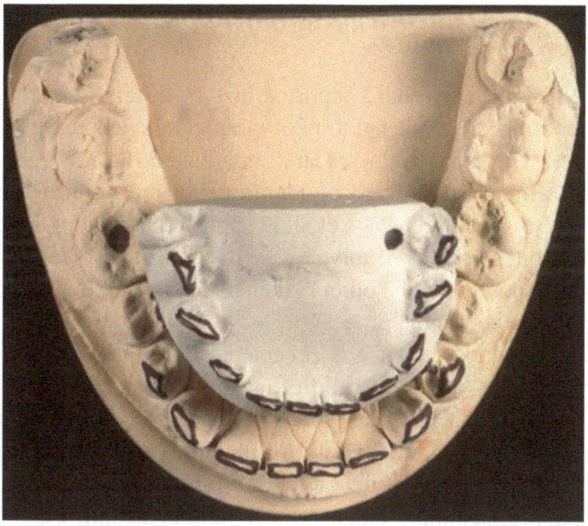

Fig. 8.4 Impression of both the deceased victim and suspect were made and transparent overlays were created

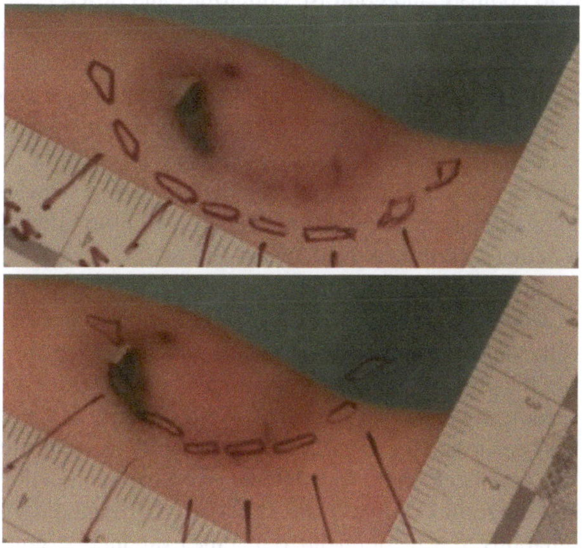

Fig. 8.5 The victim in Slide 315 demonstrating the use of transparent overlays and the ABFO scales to compare the dentitions of both the suspect and the victim with the bitemark. In this particular case, it was determined that the victim bit herself during the perimortem period

of the first signs is overall neglect of the child such as malnutrition, poor nutrition, or head lice and overall hygiene. Typically, the injury of the child occurs in the absence of another individual, or many times a sibling is blamed for the injury. It is also common that the history of injury is vague and inconsistent with clinical findings with injuries that occur in places that are away from bony prominences [18].

8.3.4 Medico-legal Implications

When an individual's reported history differs from the injury observed, mandated reporters are expected to photograph and document the suspected abuse to authorities. There has been research conducted on how reliable bitemark analysis is to informing the process of identification because of the validity and reliability of analysis methods. Page et al. [21] posit that although there is evidence that suggests that bitemark do not solve a case by themselves, the bitemark evidence must be used in the context of the other evidence that is provided and can be utilized as an adjunctive method in the process.

Bitemark evidence is accepted within the legal system, however the underpinning of its scientific validity is sometimes challenged. To increase the validity of bitemark analysis, the American Board of Forensic Odontologists (ABFO) established bitemark methodology guidelines [1]. After court orders have been issued in a case, any form of dental history prior to the bite is recorded in detail, and a front and profile photograph should be obtained along with an intra and extra oral examination. When possible, two sets of impression casts and a comprehensive dental assessment should also be completed [24]. The objective of the obtaining the casts is to compare and contrast similarities and differences between the photograph of the victim's bitemark to a scaled, digitized model of the bitemark of the suspect. After this process, it is recommended that a scoring guide that was developed by the ABFO is utilized to evaluate comparison and a conclusion made based on quantitative measure of the quality of the match based on objective measures [35]. Gupta et al. [13] that odontologists typically provide opinion to legal authorities, but do not always offer scientific reasoning behind why a conclusion was reached regarding their analysis. Sharing this reasoning will inform outside individuals about the factors that determined the decision and will serve as a source of education for others to apply to their future cases.

Courts place emphasis on evidence that has been gathered utilizing a scientifically validated approach. The court systems utilize Daubert Guidelines to standardize the use of and filter expert evidence offered to the court. Dauberts rules specifically state that in order for the evidence to be admissible, that the evidence has been tested for its evidentiary reliability. "Courts must determine if the scientific basis has been tested for trial and error, the methodological firmness of those tests, and the results of that testing" [24], p. 3. To uphold a stronger case of evidentiary reliability, it is recommended that the examiner be a qualified and experienced dental investigator, and when possible, certified by the ABFO [24].

8.4 Summary

Forensic odontology is scientifically proven to aid in the assistance of victim identification, and bitemark is utilized as and adjunctive method to assist in cases of suspected abuse. The results of certainty afforded by those efforts have satisfied matters of societal justice and given families the opportunity for needed closure [32]. Technological advancements utilized in the field of odontology will continue to grow and offer assistance to those in need. Continued education of all emergency and medical professionals is crucial for sustaining a modern process allowing for proper stewardship of evidence so that it may be utilized to its fullest potential.

References

1. American Board of Forensic Odontology. ID & Bitemark guidelines [Website]. 2013. Retrieved from http://www.abfo.org/resources/id-bitemark-guidelines/.
2. Aschheim KW, Adams B. Computerized dental coding and sorting algorithms: is there a best? J Forensic Odontostomatol. 2013;31(1):113–4. http://www.abfo.org/resources/id-bitemark-guidelines/best.
3. Bassed RB, Hill AJ. The use of computed tomography (CT) to estimate age in the 2009 Victorian bushfire victims: a case report. Forensic Sci Int. 2011;205(2011):48–51.
4. Bush MA, Miller RG, Prutsman-Pfeiffer J, Bush PJ. Identification through X-ray fluorescence analysis of dental restorative resin materials: a comprehensive study of noncremated, cremated, and processed-cremated individuals. J Forensic Sci. 2007;52(1):157–65.
5. Bush MA, Miller RG, Norrlander AL, Bush PJ. Analytical survey of restorative resins by SEM/EDS and XRF: Databases for forensic purposes. J Forensic Sci. 2008;53(2):419–25.
6. Claes P, Vandermeulen D, de Graaf S, Willems G, Clement JG, Suetens P. Review article: computerized craniofacial reconstruction: conceptual framework and review. Forensic Sci Int. 2010;201(2010):138–45.
7. Colvenkar S. Subscriber identity module: a new method for denture identification. Dent Res J (Isfahan). 2013;10(4):553–5.
8. Datta P, Sood S. The various methods and benefits of denture labeling. J Forensic Dent Sci. 2010;2(2):53–8.
9. Ebert LC, Ptacek W, Naether S, Furst M, Ross S, Buck U, Weber S, Thali M. Virtobot: a multifunctional robotic system for 3D surface scanning and automatic postmortem biopsy. Int J Med Robot Comp. 2009;6(1):18–27.
10. Flint DJ, Dove SB, Brumit PC, White M, Senn DR. Computer-aided dental identification: an objective method for assessment of radiographic image similarity. J Forensic Sci. 2009;54(1):177–84.
11. Forrest AS. Collection and recording of radiological information for forensic purposes. Aust Dent J. 2012;57(S1):24–32.
12. Franco A, Thevissen P, Coudyzer W, Dvelter W, Van de Voorde W, Oyen R, Vandermeulen D, Jacobs R, Willems G. Feasibility and validation of virtual autopsy for dental identification using Interpol dental codes. J Forensic Leg Med. 2013;20(2013):248–54.
13. Gupta A, Garg A, Chaurasia N, Datta P. Using human bite as a modern tool in forensic dentistry. Ind J Forensic Odontol. 2013;6(2):45–50.
14. Herschaft EE, editor. Manual of forensic odontology. 4th ed. Boca Raton: CRC Press Taylor & Francis Group; 2011.
15. James H, Taylor J. Australasian and multinational disaster victim identification. In: Bowers CM, editor. Dental evidence. An investigators handbook. 2nd ed. Burlington: Academic; 2011. p. 273–86.
16. Khatri M, Mariappan JD, Srinivasan SV. A comparative study of overlay generation methods in bitemark analysis. J Forensic Dent Sci. 2013;5(1):16–21.
17. Lee WJ, Wilkinson CM, Hwang HS. An accuracy assessment of forensic computerized facial reconstruction employing cone-beam computed tomography from live subjects. J Forensic Sci. 2012;57(2):318–27.

18. Mishra MN. An insight to forensic odontology and its medico-legal application. Med Leg Update. 2012;12(1):8–10.
19. National Research Council of the National Academies. Strengthening forensic science in the United States: a path forward. Washington, DC: The National Academies; 2009.
20. Nuzzolese E, Marcario V, Di Vella G. Incorporation of radio frequency identification tag in dentures to facilitate recognition and forensic human identification. Open Dent J. 2010;2010(4):33–6.
21. Page M, Taylor J, Blenkin M. Reality bites-a ten-year retrospective analysis of bitemark casework in Australia. Forensic Sci Int. 2012;216:82–7.
22. Petju M, Suteerayongprasert A, Thongpud R, Hassiri K. Importance of dental records for victim identification following the Indian Ocean tsunami disaster in Thailand. Public Health. 2007;121:251–7.
23. Pittayapat P, Oliveira-Santos C, Thevissen P, Michielsen K, Bergans N, Willems G, Debruyckere D, Jacobs R. Image quality assessment and medical physics evaluation of different portable dental x-ray units. Forensic Sci. 2010;201:112–7.
24. Rajsheker M, Kruger E, Tennant M. Bite-marks: understanding the role of general practitioners in forensic identification. J Int Oral Health. 2012;4(2):1–7.
25. Richmond R, Phil M, Pretty IA. Contemporary methods of labeling dental prostheses: a review of the literature. J Forensic Sci. 2006;51(5):1120–6.
26. Richmond R, Phil M, Pretty IA. A range of postmortem assault experiments conducted on a variety of denture labels used for the purpose of identification of edentulous individuals. J Forensic Sci. 2009;54(2):411–4.
27. Richmond R, Phil M, Pretty IA. The use of radio frequency identification tags for labeling dentures: scanning properties. J Forensic Sci. 2009;54(3):664–8.
28. Rosario AF, Souza PH, Coudyzer W, Thevissen P, Willems G, Jacobs R. Virtual autopsy in forensic sciences and its applications in forensic odontology. Rev Odonto Ciencia. 2012;271(1):5–9.
29. Rutty GN, Robinson CE, BouHaidar R, Jeffery AJ, Morgan B. The role of mobile computed tomography in mass fatality incidents. J Forensic Sci. 2007;52(6):1343–9.
30. Saxena S, Sharma P, Gupta N. Experimental studies of forensic odontology to aid in the identification process. J Forensic Dent Sci. 2010;2:69–76.
31. Senn DR, Stimson PG, editors. Forensic dentistry. 2nd ed. Boca Raton: CRC Press Taylor & Francis Group; 2010.
32. Seen DR, Weems RA, editors. Manual of forensic odontology. 5th ed. Boca Raton: CRC Press Taylor & Francis Group; 2013.
33. Shrimpton S, Daniels K, de Greef S, Tilotta F, Willems G, Vandermeulen D, Suetens P, Claes P. A spatially-dense regression study of facial form and tissue depth: towards an interactive tool for craniofacial reconstruction. Forensic Sci Int. 2014;234(2014):103–10.
34. Star H, Thevissen P, Jacobs R, Fieuws S, Solheim T, Willems G. Human dental age estimation by calculation of pulp-tooth volume ratios yielded on clinically acquired cone-beam computed tomography images of monoradicular teeth. J Forensic Sci. 2011;56(S1):S77–82.
35. Tuceryan M, Fang L, Blitzer HL, Parks ET, Platt JA. A framework for estimating probability of a match in forensic bitemark identification. J Forensic Sci. 2011;56(1):S83–9. doi:10.1111/j.1556-4029.2010.01571.x.
36. United States Department of Justice. NamUS: National Missing and Unidentified Persons System. Available at: http://www.namus.gov. Accessed 2014 Apr 19.
37. Unified Victim Identification System. UVIS information guide. Available at: http://www.nyc.gov/html/ocme/downloads/pdf/Special%20Operations/UVIS%20Information%20Guide_20090917.pdf. Accessed 2014 Apr 19.

Chapter 9
Teledentistry in Brazil

Mary Caroline Skelton-Macedo, Ana Estela Haddad, and João Humberto Antoniazzi

Abstract Teledentistry has advanced in Brazil (Numbers of Brazil – Fig. 9.1) in recent years, particularly with an emphasis on interactive teleducation, and telecare/teleassistance in the production of multicentre studies.

It is worthy to note that Brazil has adopted eHealth as a national policy applied to healthcare and education since 2006. It started as part of Ministry of Health national policy for development and capacity building of human resources for health. Many strategies have been developed and adopted aiming to reorient health professionals competencies to the healthcare model established in its universal access health system, based on primary health care. The strategies deal with undergraduate students, technical level health workers, residency and postgraduate programs. The educational policy implemented is based on three main guidelines: integration between universities and health services, a wider concept of health-disease process, based on the social determinants of health and new pedagogical approach based on active methodologies, including the use of information and communication technologies (ICT).

Keywords Unified Health System • Brazilian Telehealth Program • National Teledentistry Network • Teledentistry Centre FOUSP • Geriatric dentistry

Teledentistry has advanced in Brazil (Numbers of Brazil – Fig. 9.1) in recent years, particularly with an emphasis on interactive teleducation, and telecare/teleassistance in the production of multicentre studies.

M.C. Skelton-Macedo (✉)
Department of Dentistry-Telehealth/Teledentistry Center,
Dental School-University of São Paulo, São Paulo, Brazil
e-mail: mary@usp.br

A.E. Haddad
Department of Paediatrics, Teledentistry Centre, School of Dentistry,
University of São Paulo, São Paulo, Brazil

J.H. Antoniazzi
Department of Endodontics, Teledentistry Centre, School of Dentistry,
University of São Paulo, São Paulo, Brazil

S. Kumar (ed.), *Teledentistry*, Health Informatics,
DOI 10.1007/978-3-319-08973-7_9

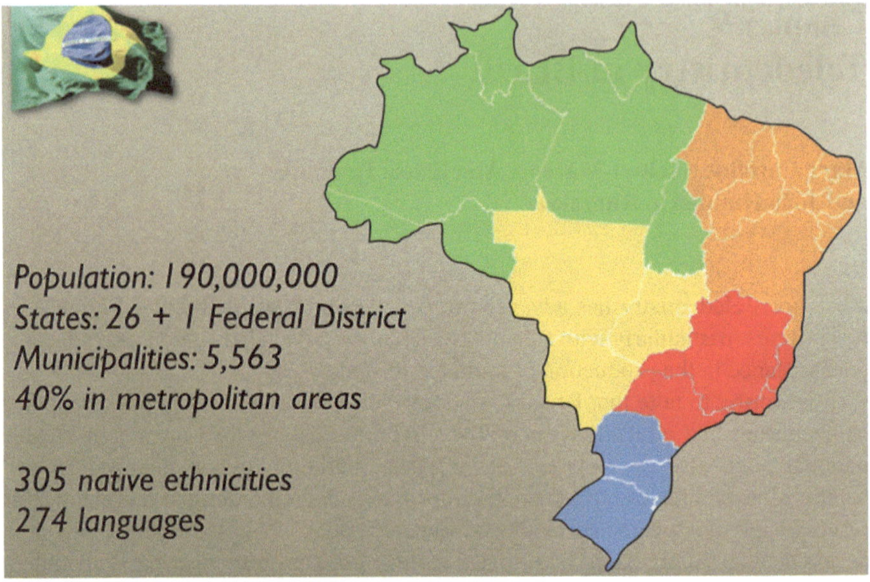

Fig. 9.1 Brazil and its numbers

It is worthy to note that Brazil has adopted eHealth as a national policy applied to healthcare and education since 2006. It started as part of Ministry of Health national policy for development and capacity building of human resources for health. Many strategies have been developed and adopted aiming to reorient health professionals competencies to the healthcare model established in its universal access health system, based on primary health care. The strategies deal with undergraduate students, technical level health workers, residency and postgraduate programs. The educational policy implemented is based on three main guidelines: integration between universities and health services, a wider concept of health-disease process, based on the social determinants of health and new pedagogical approach based on active methodologies, including the use of information and communication technologies (ICT) [1, 2].

Brazil assumed health as a right of each citizen and for that its Federal Constitution created in 1988 the Unified Health System (SUS), which applies currently to more than 190 million inhabitants. One of the greatest challenges faced by universal health systems is how deal with the overpowering increase of new technologies applied to healthcare and, at the same time, guarantee universal access of population to high quality of care with sustainability. Human health resources play a central hole in this equation [3].

A special issue number of the Lancet with a series of papers about the Unified Health System (SUS) from Brazil was published in 2011. As far as the Millenium Development Goals – MDG are concerned, the editors highlight SUS achievements as the reduction of 50 % in low birth weight and two thirds decrease in infant mortality in the last decade [4, 5].

In this context, where we have SUS and more recently a national policy for human health resources, is that Brazilian eHealth strategies emerged and have been developed [4, 6–12].

The multiple strategies for eHealth include mainly the Brazilian Telehealth Program (www.telessaudebrasil.org.br) [13], Open University of the Unified National Health System – UNA SUS (www.unasus.gov.br) [14] and Telemedicine University Network – RUTE (www.rute.rnp.br) [15]. The activities grew faster between physicians and nurses. It has also a great acceptance and demand by Health Community Workers.

Dentistry has gained strength within SUS in 2000, when the dentists starting to integrate Family Health Teams at the primary health care level, and also with the creation of the Centers of Dental Specialties in 2005. By 2012 we reached approximately 18.000 out of 32.000 Family Health Teams that included dentists and 800 Centers of Dental Specialties all over the country. Until that most of the population had difficulties to dental treatment access. Epidemiological studies comparing the situation in 2000 and 2010 showed considerable improvement in dental health indicators, although we still have a great cumulative demand accumulated along many years before, especially in relation to adult oral health needs.

This active inclusion of Dentistry within SUS created the necessity for undergraduate programs to prepare better students to a new professional activity pattern, facing the challenge of working in a multiprofessional team, at public services and not only in private offices. Many programs and strategies are being promoted by the federal Government, specially by the Ministries of Health, of Education and of Science, Technology and Innovation to face the new challenges involving all health professionals, including dentists.

One of them is the eHealth strategy and to better integrate Dentistry [16, 17], it was created the National Teledentistry Network – RNTO (http://programa.telessaudebrasil.org.br/vhl/teleodontologia-em-foco/rede-nacional-de-teleodontologia-e-nucleos) in 2011 (Fig. 9.2). Its goal is to share and exchange successful experiences of telehealth applied to teledentistry, nationally and abroad. Two relevant RNTO initiatives must be mentioned. One of them is the e-learning course destined to institutions interested in developing Teledentistry Centers. It is divided in three modules: (*1*) *How to implement and manage a Teledentistry Center;* (*2*) *How to train and stimulate professors to use more widely information and communication technologies (ICT) in the teaching-learning process;* (*3*) *How to support a service of teleconsultancies and Formative Second Opinion for health professionals.* Each module has been structured by experienced professors and dentists already engaged on Brazilian Telehealth Program [13] and UNA SUS [14], establishing guidelines and learned lessons that may help new partners to better perform in the network. After defining the content and validating it by an experienced external committee, the module is developed with the support of a instructional design that has a pedagogical background. It is expected that this course may serve as a reference for teachers, health professionals, faculties of Dentistry and health services willing to start using ICT for teaching and learning and healthcare support.

The second initiative, as part of RUTE [15], is the creation of a Special Interest Group (SIG) in Teledentistry (Fig. 9.3). It represents one, out of more than 40 SIGs

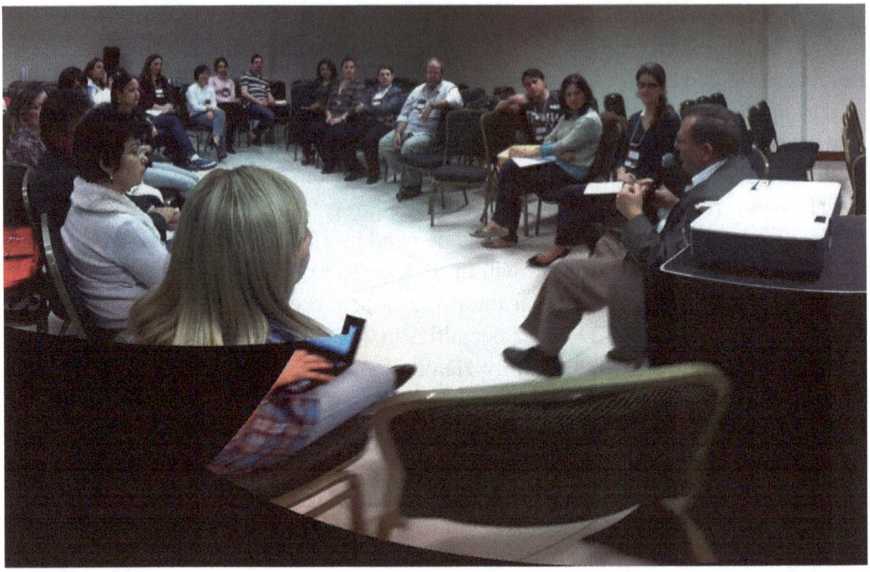

Fig. 9.2 Launch of the National Network of Teledentistry with eight colleges/states represented, 2011 – Santa Catarina, Brazil

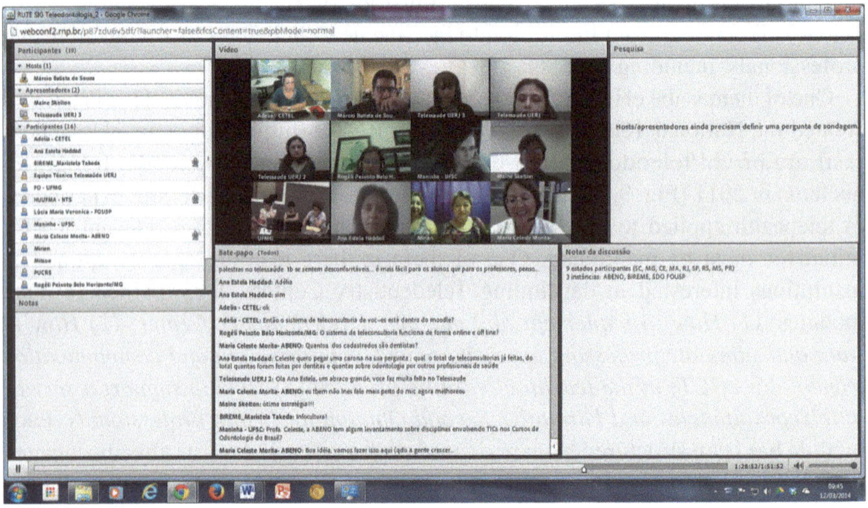

Fig. 9.3 Teledentistry Special Interest Group – monthly meeting, at RUTE – Telemedicine University Network

already at work, in different specialties most of them in Medicine and Nursery. The Teledentistry SIG is a virtual space in which education and research institutions from all over the country get together virtually through video and web conference, discuss, share their experience and learn how to better work as an effectively connected network. This huge movement of education and research in health network was made possible by a cooperative initiative run by the Ministry of Science and Technology, with partnership with the Ministries of Education and of Health. A backbone of wide band has been built connecting all the public university hospitals and other relevant health services, connecting this national wide network dedicated to education and research in health field. There is a Social Organization, the National Network of Education and Research (www.rnp.br) [18], from the Ministry of Science and Technology, which is responsible for the development and management of RUTE.

The RNTO is run by the Brazilian Association of Dental Education (www.abeno.org.br) [19] and by the Teledentistry Center of the Faculty of Dentistry of University of Sao Paulo (www.teleodonto.fo.usp.br) [20], in partnership with the Telehealth Centers of the University of the State of Rio de Janeiro – UERJ (http://www.telessaude.uerj.br) [21], Federal University of Rio Grande do Sul – UFRGS (http://www.ufrgs.br/telessauders) [22] and the State Secretary of Health of Mato Grosso do Sul (http://telessaude.saude.ms.gov.br) [23]. The project is supported by the Ministry of Health (www.saude.gov.br) [24] with the cooperation of Pan American Health Organization (PAHO) [25]. The two initiatives are articulated and their effects on the function, strengthen and extension of the RNTO. It has also contributed for the improvement of healthcare, research and education in undergraduate and pos graduate dentistry courses all over the country.

The tools of Telehealth and Teledentistry allow break through the limits of the geographical and temporal distance, so that professionals, whether working in remote areas, have access to communication with other centers and services, no longer feel isolated (Fig. 9.4).

Nowadays, whatever the diagnosis or health problem presented, there is a tendency of the population, with growing access to the Internet, to search for knowledge about their own condition. We must seize this window of opportunity to guide the search for quality information and credibility. It is important that professionals are prepared to take these guidelines as well as to be a source of reliable information about health promotion and prevention in relation to general health and oral health.

The first decade of the twenty-first century can be considered the starting point of the first Brazilian initiative in Teledentistry. Many distance-learning courses were produced in Brazil. It began with the concern of informing patients and professionals, for instance, about oral cancer [26].

The Department of FMUSP's Telemedicine [27], which had already worked with telemedicine connections across Brazil, developed modules related to Dental Health. In the *São Paulo Center* that is linked to Brazils National Telehealth Program [13], a platform is used supporting continuous education for professionals working in primary health care. One of the projects being developed is the *Virtual Human* involving human anatomical and physiological aspects in 3D animation, with various titles related to dentistry, for instance: *Temporomandibular Joint* (TMJ), Dental Structure (2004); *Anaesthesia in Paediatric Dentistry and tooth extraction of deciduous teeth (2011)*; *Development of dental caries; and traumatic lesions* (2007–2009) *ATM and Dysfunctions* (2008); *Oral Health in the Elderly* (2008).

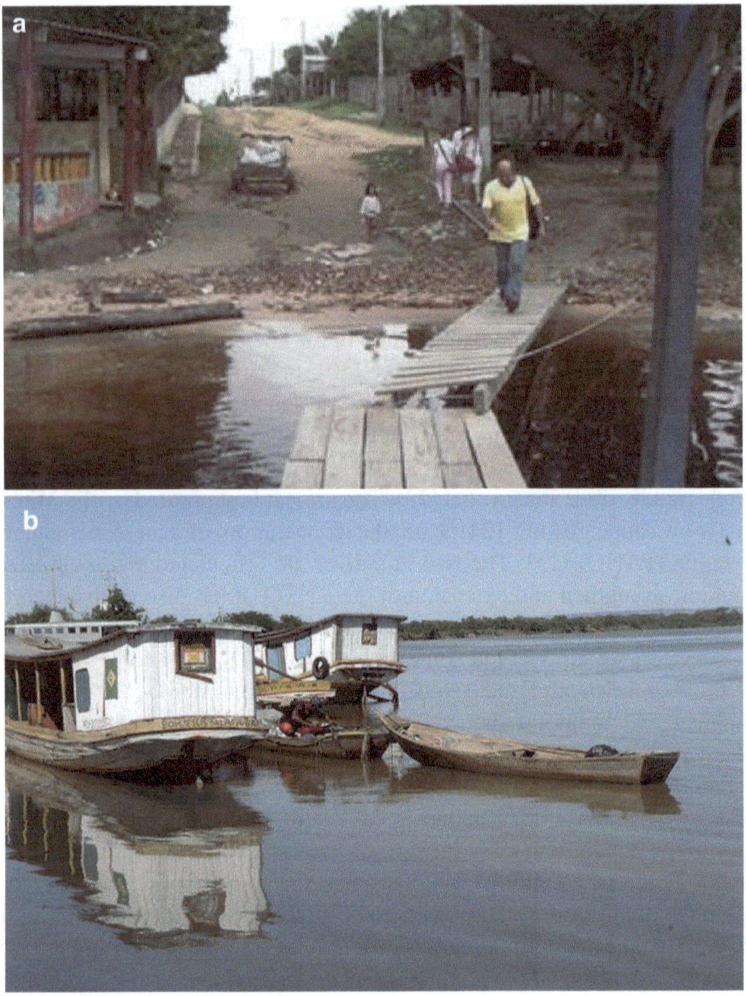

Fig. 9.4 (**a**) Geographic problems to access people – State of Minas Gerais. (**b**) Geographic problems to access people – State of Amazonas

These results led the USP team to participate in the planning and implementation of the Brazil Telehealth Network [13] program in 2006, in conjunction with the Brazilian Ministry of Health.

In Telecare, through collaboration with USP and USC, the development of Dental Telepropaedeutics was initiated, with the creation of online clinical records and educational lectures about drug interaction, the *International Classification of Diseases* (ICD), references, educational reports, epidemiologic data, and other [27]

The first and second Brazilian Meetings of Teledentistry were organized within the Congress of Brazilian Council for Telemedicine and Telehealth (CBTms) [28], resulting in a consensus document: Consensus Belo Horizonte [29], Minas Gerais – Brazil:

> The dissemination of Teledentistry in Brazil is important to improve the quality of education, for this reason, the creation of Teledentistry centres of Higher Education Institutions (HEIs) should be encouraged along with the training of new professionals. The educational institutions, regulation and standard of Dentistry will ensure the appropriate use of technology in teaching, research and additional development.
>
> Dentistry has an important role in the health of the Brazilian population. With the help of Teledentistry, institutions and university groups can promote national stimulus programs for oral health, and the possibility of partnerships between public, private and non-governmental organizations (NGOs) and agencies.
>
> The modernization of educational iconography, through the development of learning tools should be considered as a strategic action to improve the quality of education in dentistry. It is important to join the Dental Front Pro-FUST (Fund for Universalization of Telecommunications Services) through the Department of Teledentistry of CBTMs and dental education articles. This section of dentistry is design for the release of funds from the FUST to be used in education and health.
>
> It is necessary to prepare the regulation for the use of Teledentistry among professionals and professional-patient relationship.
>
> The promotion of Brazilian Teledentistry at the 10th International Telemedicine Congress, which was held in October 2005 in São Paulo, was appropriate.
>
> Collaborating Teledentistry centres should be encouraged amongst HEIs for the sharing of projects and experiences in teaching, research and extensions.

The 25th International Dental Congress in 2007 discussed the ethics of Teledentistry and Distance Education. The debate allowed participants to clarify questions about the use of ICT (Information and Communication), with the emphasis on professional – patient relationship, the teaching and learning process, and the teacher-student relationship.

Torres-Pereira et al. [30], of the Federal University of Paraná (UFPR) studied images sent via e-mail to test the accuracy of lesions of the oral mucosa diagnosis. Twenty-five cases were documented in 12 months in the primary care health service. The images were sent to two experts in Semiology with over 10 years' experience. In 88 % of cases, at least one of the experts made the correct diagnosis. The authors conclude that Teledentistry can be a viable alternative for the diagnosis of oral mucosal lesions in remote locations and primary care services when there are no experts available in Semiology.

Skelton-Macedo and Antoniazzi [31] reflected on the benefits of ICT for professional discussions. The importance of a second opinion in geographically isolated areas was observed; as well as the ethical issues related to professional responsibility for the care they provided, reliability, confidentiality of information in circulation and the importance of regulating the use of Teledentistry.

In his PhD thesis, Abranches [32] developed and evaluated an educational website for the prevention of oral cancer. Most cases are diagnosed late and self-examination is a simple and effective measure in the early diagnosis of precancerous lesions and oral cancer. It was concluded that the website had proven to be an effective educational tool with regards to the increasing of personal knowledge on the subject of oral cancer and provided a tool for effective repeatable oral self-examination. She also submitted his website to HON – Health on the Net Foundation (www.hon.ch) and received a certification seal.

9.1 The Teledentistry Centre FOUSP School of Dentistry, University of São Paulo

In 2000, the Discipline of General Pathology (graduation) build a website which provided innovative educational content and material to support classroom learning and initiatives for distance learning [33].

Department of Endodontics (undergraduate) made a CD with the contents of Endodontic Technique FOUSP, in 2002.

Parallel to these experiments, two disciplines: Dental Educational Methodology and Research Methodology (post-graduation) incorporated the application of educational technologies in 2004, supporting classroom content using virtual learning environments – AVA (TelEduc – UNICAMP, CoL – USP and Moodle). Asynchronous and synchronous communication tools have been applied and the impressions of professors and students were collected, which showed that the new forms of communication support the classroom teaching significantly altering the teacher-student relationship and provide better student involvement in the learning process (since 1998).

Some subjects/disciplines felt compelled to start their own projects on the use of technological innovations in 2007, such as occurred with the Discipline of Dentistry (Graduation). It was designed new ways to build educational resources, involving Augmented Reality (a PhD thesis, which received the Edmir Matson Award in 2011) [34].

The invitation for the establishment of a Centre for Teledentistry FOUSP at the beginning of 2007 came from SGTES (Management Secretariat of Labour and Health Education, Ministry of Health) to integrate the São Paulo Telehealth core. It added the University initiatives and developed expertise with new standards and requirements related to the possibility of issuing a second opinion for public health service professionals, expanding the line of action beyond Teleducation, also working as Telecare Professionals. Profs Antoniazzi JH (Chairman of Endodontics discipline) and Guedes-Pinto AC (Chairman of Paediatric Dentistry) were invited to coordinate the process of building this new science at the school.

The Centres for Telehealth and Teledentistry are defined as spaces constituted by HEIs, with multidisciplinary technical and pedagogical teams, having as its main objectives:

- To support the faculty and students in developing skills and competencies in the information and communication technologies (ICT) usage as applied to teaching, research and healthcare.
- Supporting the teaching-services multidisciplinary health teamwork by examining the demand of teleconsultations and the cataloguing of Formative Second Opinions.

Primary Care Dental Health issue was to updated (available in Portuguese, English and Spanish) [35].

Two postdoctoral students conducted their work focused on the actions of the Centre: supporting Telecare actions, with the establishment of a Telehealth unit in a Basic Health Unit and organizing the Discipline of Telehealth and Teledentistry for undergraduate students (Development and implementation of the Teledentistry discipline and Reference Centre for Development of Teaching Materials FOUSP). The centre also responsible for structuring the production of educational material, incorporating a mini studio, a living thesis presentation room, that connected professor to participate from remote locations, and digital classroom. It is the first Teledentistry Centre structured in the country.

From these innovative experiences, the Department of Paediatric Dentistry initiated a training program for post-graduation students to be guardians of undergraduate students, incorporating new skills for the teaching of master degree students, in 2008. With the development of educational material: Virtual Human in *Evaluation of the contents and the learning object in Teledentistry applied to anaesthesia and extraction in Paediatric Dentistry* [36] and *Design and evaluation of an extension course in Atraumatic Restorative Treatment* (ART) *using distance education* [37], made it possible to reach new applications and working partnerships using 3D animation, developed by the Department of Telemedicine USP (School of Medicine, University of São Paulo) (Fig. 9.5).

An analysis of the legal aspects regulating the exchange of sensitive data was conducted by the Centre, to inform the dangers of a communication, which may expose the confidentiality of relevant information of patients. In 2008, a regulatory document was developed and submitted to the Federal Council of Dentistry (CFO) [38].

The Discipline of Telehealth and Teledentistry was developed and offered to graduation and post-graduation students, giving them the opportunity to develop projects of citizenship action, facilitated by educational technologies geared for different application contexts (awareness campaigns; educational material development; mapping cultural opportunities given by the University; among others). The applied strategy is to learn by projects in which students are exposed to the benefits that technology can produce, changing realities in the social and healthcare context. The results are very interesting, from projects aimed at student reception at the university to mobile applications that protect caregivers with special needs.

Other disciplines started their activities with digital content, like Bioethics [39], Prosthetics and Periodontology. The response from students was total involvement and a depth of learning.

The initiatives mentioned above raised important issues that had to be mapped and studied in order to meet the demands of the country's dental surgeons in order to continually improving the quality of dental care offered in Brazil. This led Professor Ana Estela Haddad to coordinate a national survey project, published in January 2010 under the title Current Profile and Trends of the Brazilian Dental Surgeon, which gathers important data on the distribution of dental surgeons and allows a larger view of the needs of education and care of the professional [7].

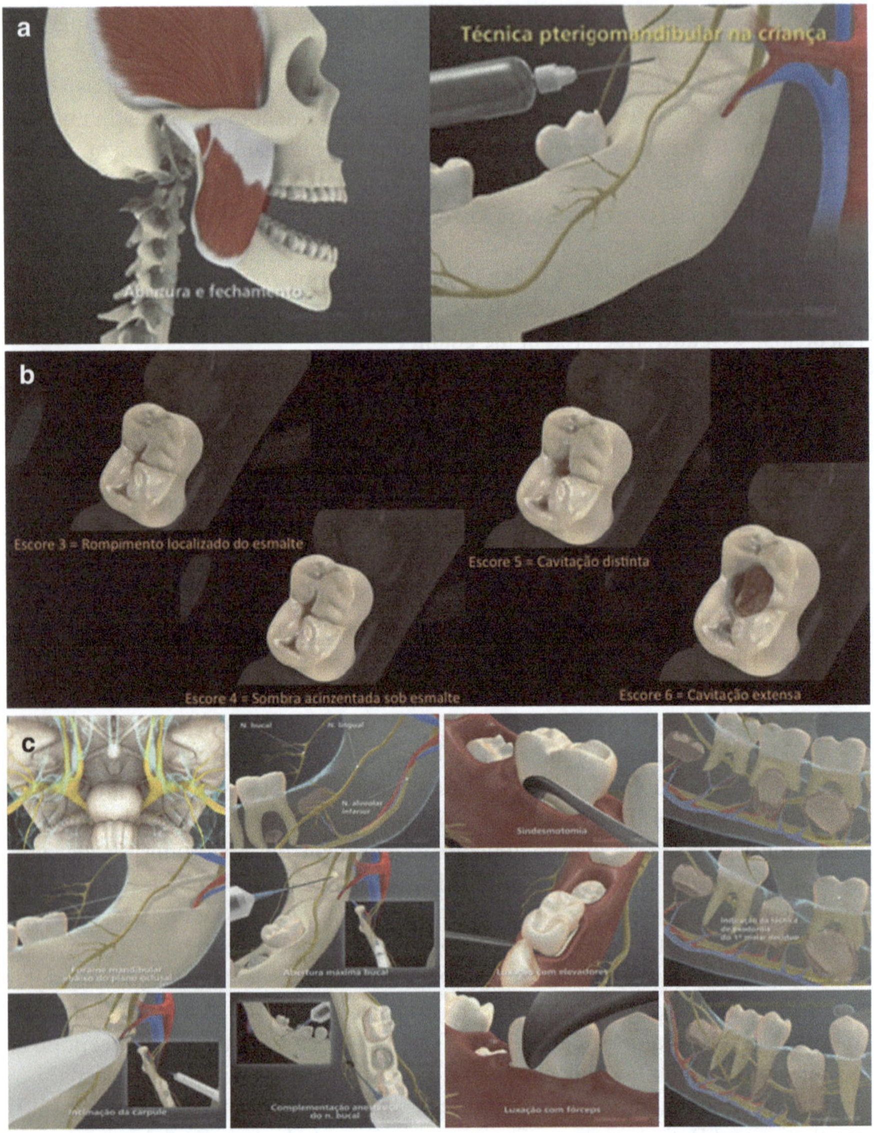

Fig. 9.5 (**a–c**) Images from three thesis, built on 3D animation, called Virtual Man – FMUSP, Brazil

These actions concluded with the FOUSP hiring the first Teledentistry professor and a technician in order to support the demand in a productive and efficient manner in 2010. During the probation period, Prof. Mary Caroline Skelton–Macedo, under the coordination of Prof. João Humberto Antoniazzi and Professor Ana Estela Haddad, created a National Network of Teledentistry that would involve Teledentistry initiatives in the country. It would also integrate the National Telehealth Program of the

Ministry of Health, and making relevant actions through Telecare in Dentistry meeting the specific needs of this area of knowledge. This project was presented to the Ministry of Health [23]/PAHO [24], bringing valuable resources to the school and enabling the integration of Teledentistry in the Open University of SUS (UNA-SUS) [13], along with ObservRHodonto Network (first observatory of Dental Staff of the country) [10].

Some of the Telehealth Centres in the country have developed Teledentistry activities: Amazonas, Pernambuco, Maranhão, Rio de Janeiro, Rio Grande do Sul, Mato Grosso do Sul, Minas Gerais and Goiás.

The Teledentistry field of the Federal University of Maranhão (UFMA), in partnerships with USP and UERJ, has developed Extension Courses for self-instructional Dentistry with different subjects. These courses will also be available in the form of applications of UNASUS [13]/UFMA or HEI partners that enable the offline study by mobile responsive technology, which was first used by UFMA in UNASUS Network [13]. There will be thousands of vacancies for courses as it does not need to be mediated by mentors and will be available allow free access to the partner universities' platforms as applications. At the end of the course, SAD (Document Authentication System) will provide a certification.

Another successful experience at UFMA was the offering of the ODL course in Geriatric dentistry for Masters and PhD students of the Graduate Program in Dentistry. The focus of the course was Primary Care and provided rich forum discussions, which led to a fruitful opportunity for students to use their academic knowledge in the SUS practice. The students were so pleased with the experience that they requested more courses with this methodology, not only in PPGO/UFMA program, but also in other healthcare post-graduation course in the Institution.

Still within the Telehealth Networks Program, the National Network of Teledentistry already has some of its items integrating the APS – VHL (Virtual Health Library in Primary Care), in the form of Formative Second Opinions (questions sent to the core of Telehealth and generated structured responses, based on clinical and scientific evidence presented in the form of questions and answers on the program page) [12]. Currently the library has approximately 700 questions and answers, of which approximately 20 % are dental issues. It was raised some interesting information such as: from the 134 Second Opinions on Oral Health topics, the most referred were subthemes such as: Paediatric Dentistry, followed by general practice, Patients with Special needs, Surgery and Traumatology, Pharmacology, Semiology, Endodontic, Periodontics and Oral Health Education. The least required were Public Health and Orthodontics. Within each subject, an associated subtheme was traced in paediatric Dentistry and general practice. There were a wide range of subjects involving dental questions and dental surgeons were responsible for most of these questions. There were two questions about Dentistry made by Physicians; two questions made by oral health assistant; four questions were made by the Community Health; and one question made by a Nurse. Although there is little information on this subject, it is possible to verify that other healthcare professionals are interested in this subject. The low usage of the program could be related to the fact that the dental surgeons joined the Family Health Strategy more recently (in 2000, with the creation of Oral Health Teams). New projects have been designed in order to increase professional involvement as the program offers clinical decision support with qualified information.

The experiments cited drew attention to educational applications in the virtual context, which allows us to resize the classroom and to deliver an investigative content that is more closely related to real life context currently experienced by young students. Such students are seamlessly integrated in the ICT in their day -to-day activities. What is noticeable is that teachers have much greater resistance to the incorporation of ICT than the students, who already make many uses of these innovations and easily understand their educational application. The concept of innovation needs to be understood: the technology is innovative to those born before it, not so for those who were born after the *innovation* who incorporated this technology into their daily lives, which encourages its use in various fields. The professors difficulties are plausible, but it is noted here that the more they engage with these applications, the more importance and comprehension there will be about the concept of citizenship and ethics in the digital scope, facilitating learning and enhancing aspects such as access to education, optimization, streamlining of processes and modification of educational realities in the healthcare context.

In 2011 the Centre build the National Network Teledentistry [20]: Integration with Telehealth Programs in Brazil, UnA – SUS [14] and Observarhodonto Network, the Ministry of Health/PAHO [25], at the Management of Health Education Department (DEGES), the Work management department and Health Education (SGTES) for the development of resources and training courses for tutors for the Open University Programs SUS (Unified Health System) – UNA-SUS [14] – and Telehealth, for the development by the Observatory Network. In the same period, there was a partnership with the School of Medicine of the USP by the National Coordination for the Improvement of Higher Education of the Ministry of Education (CAPES/MEC), titled Interactive Educational Technologies for potentiation of Health Education, obtaining resources for infrastructure and development of broader significance for Education in Health.

At present, the Centre integrates a discussion for open access content, according to the principles of *International Open Access movement*. In this way, FOUSP is developing a repository for educational resources. We study the policy of implementing the use and reprocess of educational material developed in the Faculty, as well as a policy of Copyright and Intellectual Property, securing to authors a greater number of citations and reuse of the material developed by them, increasing the importance of professors' work in the production of educational resources. Because of this action, the Centre integrates the study group for construction of software repositories at the University, with the SIBi (Integrated Library System USP).

There are currently over 100 courses hosted in the Teledentistry centre Moodle, involving spaces used for Undergraduate Courses, Postgraduate, Extension, added to the spaces used by Undergraduate and Graduate students to support the work of the Interdisciplinary assembly and independent studies groups.

Hopefully training teachers with the use of ICT, we can train students to understand the use of electronic tools to improve the health of populations, with innovations of use and applications.

References

1. Haddad AE. A Odontologia na Política de Formação dos Profissionais de Saúde, o papel da Teleodontologia como ferramenta do processo de ensino-aprendizagem e a criação do Núcleo de Teleodontologia da FOUSP. Tese de Livre-Docência. Faculdade de Odontologia da USP. 2011. 198p. Available at http://www.teses.usp.br/teses/disponiveis/livredocencia/23/tde-13052013-143506/pt-br.php. Accessed Jan 2014.
2. Kleinert S, Horton R. Brazil: towards sustainability and equity in health. Lancet. 2011; 377(9779):1721–2.
3. Haddad AE. Brazilian Experience in Telehealth Brazil Program. In: Gold Book 50° Congresso Científico do HUPE. eBook. Tecnologia em Educação e Saúde. 2012. Available at www.telessaude.uerj.br/goldbook/artigos. Accessed Jan 2014.
4. Bradley M, Black P, Noble R, Thompson R, Lamey PJ. Application of teledentistry in oral medicine in a community dental service, Northern Ireland. Br Dent J. 2010;209(8):399–404.
5. Haddad AE, Skelton-Macedo MC, Castro EDFo, Abdala CV, Andrade RMP, Campos FE. Formative second opinion: qualifying primary health care in Brazil. Global Telemed eHealth Updates: Knowledge Resources. 2010;3:546–50.
6. Gundim RS, Chao LW. A graphical representation model for telemedicine and telehealth center sustainability. Telemed J E Health. 2011;17(3):164–8.
7. World Health Organization. WHA 58.28 Resolution of 2005. Available at http://apps.who.int/iris/bitstream/10665/20378/1/WHA58_28-en.pdf. Accessed Jan 2014.
8. Morita MC, Haddad AE, Araújo ME. Perfil atual e tendências do cirurgião-dentista brasileiro. Maringá: Editora Dental Press; 2010. 96p, Available at http://cfo.org.br/wp-content/uploads/2010/04/PERFIL_CD_BR_web.pdf.
9. Morita MC. Experiências exitosas na saúde fortalecem o ensino. Rev ABENO. 2011;11(1):5.
10. Haddad AE, Peres MA, Morita MC, Opperman RV, Moyses SJ. Pesquisa odontológica no Brasil e sua articulação com as políticas públicas de saúde. Rev Espaço para a Saúde. 2008;9(2):47–53. Available at www.ccs.uel.br/espacoparasaude/v9n2/Relato%20de%20Experincia.pdf. Accessed Jan 2014.
11. Global Observatory in Health. Available at www.who.int/goe/en. Accessed Jan 2014.
12. Organization Regional Office for the Americas. Strategy for improving general health in the Americas through critical advancements in oral health – the way forward: 2005–2015. Washington, DC: Pan American Health Organization; 2005. Available at http://new.paho.org/hq/dmdocuments/2009/OH_StratMovFWD2005-2015Eng-2.pdf.
13. Telessaúde Brasil Redes – Telehealth Brazilian Network Program. Available at www.telessaude.org.br. Accessed Jan 2014.
14. UNASUS – Open University of Brazilian Unified Health System. Available at www.unasus.gov.br. Accessed Jan 2014.
15. Rede Universitária de Telessaúde – Telehealth University Network. Available at https://rute.rnp.br. Accessed Jan 2014.
16. Ministry of Health, Brazil. Edict n.2.546 de October 27th 2011. Increases the coverage and the scope of the Brazilian Telehealth Program from PHC to the entire network of SUS. Available at http://bvsms.saude.gov.br/bvs/saudelegis/gm/2011/prt2546_27_10_2011.html. Accessed Jan 2014.
17. World Health Organization. Global Observatory for e-Health. 2005. Available at http://www.who.int/goe/en/. Accessed Jan 2014.
18. RNP Brazilian Network of Teaching and Research. Available at www.rnp.br. Accessed Jan 2014.
19. Associação Brasileira do Ensino Odontológico – Brazilian Association for Dental Teaching – ABENO. Available at www.abeno.org.br. Accessed Jan 2014.
20. Núcleo de Teleodontologia FOUSP – Teledentistry Centre of Dental School – University of São Paulo, Brazil. Available at www.teleodonto.fo.usp.br/nucleo. Accessed on Jan 2014.
21. Telehealth at University of Rio de Janeiro State. Available at www.telessaude.uerj.br/site Accessed Jan 2014.

22. Telehealth at Federal University of Rio Grande do Sul. Available at www.ufrgs.br/telessauders. Accessed Jan 2014.
23. Telehealth at Mato Grosso do Sul State. Available at http://telessaude.saude.ms.gov.br/portal. Accessed Jan 2014.
24. Brazilian Ministry of Health. Available at www.saude.gov.br. Accessed Jan 2014.
25. Panamerican Health Organization. Available at www.paho.org. Accessed Jan 2014.
26. Menendez-Castillero ME, Skelton-Macedo MC. Oral cancer prevention. Available at www.espacoabertto.com.br/cabucal/index.html. Accessed Jan 2014.
27. Estação Médica Digital – Medical Digital Station. Available at www.estacaodigitalmedica.com.br/teleodontoct. Accessed Jan 2014.
28. Conselho Brasileiro de Telemedicina e Telessaúde – Brazilian Council for Telemedicine and Telehealth. Available at www.cbtms.org.br. Accessed Jan 2014.
29. Consensus of Belo Horizonte MG. Available at www.cbtms.org.br/departamento/teleodontologia/consensoBH.html. Accessed Jan 2014.
30. Torres-Pereira C, Posselon RS, Simões A, Bortoluzzi MC, Leão JC, Giovanini F, et al. Email for distance diagnosis of oral disease: a preliminary study of teledentistry. J Telemed Telecare. 2008;14:435–8.
31. Macedo-Skelton MC, Antoniazzi JH. The benefits and newly required practices brought about by innovations in the communication between professionals. Braz Oral Res. 2009;23(2):99–100.
32. Abranches DC. Prevenção do câncer bucal: desenvolvimento e avaliação de um website educacional [tese de Doutorado]. Universidade Federal de São Paulo; 2010. Available at www.dominiopublico.gov.br/pesquisa/DetalheObraForm.do?select_action=&co_obra=196570. Accessed Jan 2014.
33. Corrêa L. Análise da mudança de paradigma do ensino de graduação em patologia na odontologia: proposta de ensino-aprendizado à distância via internet [tese]. Universidade de São Paulo: Faculdade de Odontologia; 2001. Available at http://www.teses.usp.br/teses/disponiveis/23/23141/tde-23042007-155640/pt-br.php. Accessed Jan 2014.
34. Espejo-Trung LC. Elaboração e aplicação de um novo objeto de aprendizagem para o ensino de preparo cavitário em Dentística – introdução da realidade aumentada. Available at www.teses.usp.br/teses/disponiveis/23/23134/tde-13042013-122117/pt-br.php. Accessed Jan 2014.
35. Brazilian Primary Health Notebooks – Dental Health. Available at http://issuu.com/teleodonto. Accessed Jan 2014.
36. Alencar CJF. Avaliação de conteúdos e objeto de aprendizagem da Teleodontologia aplicado a anestesia e exodontia em Odontopediatria. Available at www.teses.usp.br/teses/disponiveis/23/23132/tde-28042009-115111/pt-br.php. Accessed Jan 2014.
37. Camargo LB. Estruturação e avaliação de curso de extensão em Tratamento Restaurador Atraumático (ART) utilizando a educação a distância. Available at www.teses.usp.br/teses/disponiveis/23/23132/tde-22122010-121118/pt-br.php. Accessed Jan 2014.
38. Skelton-Macedo MC, Jacob CH, Haddad AE, Ramos DLP, Cardoso RJA, Antoniazzi JH. Contribuição para a regulamentação da conduta ética na utilização de registros eletrônicos odontológicos (REO). Available at http://www.sbpqo.org.br/arquivos/REGULAMENTACAO%20versao%207%20BOR.pdf. Accessed Jan 2014.
39. Puplaksis N. A contribuição da bioética para a formação dos profissionais da saúde de odontologia. Available at www.teses.usp.br/teses/disponiveis/23/23148/tde-20012009-150128/pt-br.php. Accessed Jan 2014.

Chapter 10
Teleconsultation and Telediagnosis for Oral Health Assessment: An Australian Perspective

Rodrigo Mariño, K. Clarke, D.J. Manton, A. Stranieri, R. Collmann, H. Kellet, and A. Borda

Abstract Oral health informatics is the application of Information and Communication Technology (ICT) for problem solving complex and dynamic information and system interactions in dental science and oral health, research and education.

In the last few years, there has been rapid development and expansion of the uses of Information and Communication Technology (ICT) and it is presently used in many areas of oral health care practice. ICT offers new opportunities to improve oral health care by enhancing early diagnosis, facilitating timely treatment of oral diseases, and reducing isolation of practitioners through communication with peers and consultation with specialists. Above all, ICT offers improved access to care as an effective alternative to classic face-to-face oral health professional-patient interaction, in terms of both clinical results and cost-effectiveness. Still, compared to medicine, teledentistry is rarely used in everyday oral health practice.

R. Mariño (✉) • D.J. Manton
Principal, Research Fellow, Oral Health Cooperative Research Centre,
Melbourne Dental School, The University of Melbourne,
Melbourne, VIC 3010, Australia
e-mail: rmarino@unimelb.edu.au

K. Clarke
Institute for a Broadband-Enabled Society, University of Melbourne, Melbourne, Australia
e-mail: clak@unimelb.edu.au

A. Stranieri
Centre for Informatics and Applied Optimisation, University of Ballarat, Ballarat, Australia
e-mail: a.stranieri@ballarat.edu.au

R. Collmann
Victorian eResearch Strategic Initiative, University of Melbourne, Melbourne, Australia
e-mail: rcollmann@unimelb.edu.au

H. Kellet
Royal Children's Hospital Melbourne, Melbourne, Australia
e-mail: kerrod.hallett@rch.org.au

A. Borda
Health and Biomedical Informatics Centre, Melbourne Medical School,
University of Melbourne, Melbourne, Australia
e-mail: aborda@unimelb.edu.au

S. Kumar (ed.), *Teledentistry*, Health Informatics,
DOI 10.1007/978-3-319-08973-7_10

This chapter reviews developments in teledentistry, outlines the benefits of applications in teledentistry and provides information on the rationale for the use of teledentistry. A second part provides an overview of teledentistry and its uses in different scenarios based on experiences in various research projects in the areas of teleconsultation and telediagnosis in Australia. These are projects that represent responses to the serious dental workforce shortage in underserved Australian communities and are equally applicable to many countries facing the same issue.

Keywords Residential aged care facility • Intra-oral camera • Periodontal examination • General dental practitioners • Cleft lip and palate • Plain Language Statement

10.1 Introduction

The concept of teledentistry involves the application of a variety of information and communications technologies (ICT) to facilitate and extend oral healthcare for patients who are physically located at another site from the oral health professional. The application of teledentistry suggests a range of possible beneficial applications, such as the efficient delivery of health records, improved communication between providers and patients, and enhanced education opportunities [6, 8, 21]. Today's high resolution and reliable digital and online technology facilitates connectivity for remote oral health promotion, education, and assessment.

Despite the fact that telemedicine has been in use for over 30 years: for consultation, diagnosis and treatment in a broad range of medical fields, there has been little use of similar ICT-focused practices within the dental profession [17]. Notwithstanding the relatively slow adoption of teledentistry in recent decades, the implementation of teledentistry is increasing, most notably in the United States and Europe [18]. Teledentistry has the potential to enhance dental care through early diagnosis, facilitating timely treatment of oral diseases, reducing isolation of practitioners through communication with peers and consultation with specialists, and by improving access to care. It also addresses the practitioners' increasing demand for distance learning, as well as oral health promotion and health education of the population. If the practice of teledentistry parallels that of telemedicine, people living in rural or under-served areas are among those that will benefit most from ICT usage in dentistry [2, 4]. For example, regional and remote Australia has major oral health workforce shortages, in particular, oral health specialists (i.e. oral pathologist, special needs dentist). Teledentistry also provides the opportunity for the primary care practitioner to be involved in the oral diagnosis and development of the treatment plan for distant patients [11].

The potential of teledentistry is vast, however a significant shortcoming of the current oral health system is its failure to take advantage of innovations in health promotion and e-technologies to influence how people assume more responsibility for their own oral health. This failure is also impacted by the paucity of research informing oral health practices and identifying innovative ways to utilise ehealth and mhealth to make both preventative and care intervention programs more accessible, particularly for those living in rural Australia.

In this chapter developments in oral health informatics are reviewed; the benefits and rationale for the use of teledentistry identified and outlined. A second part provides an overview of teledentistry and its use in different scenarios based on experiences in various research projects in the areas of teleconsultation and telediagnosis, created as responses to the serious dental workforce shortage in Australia. The described project targeted underserved, high-risk populations with great oral health care needs to assess whether improvements in accessibility and appropriateness of oral health services can be achieved by using ICT to screen for oral health problems.

10.2 Benefits of Teledentistry

As the capability of ICT has risen, a wide range of possible beneficial applications in different fields have emerged [6, 8, 10]. Expanded use of ICT has provided dental clinicians with alternatives to the traditional face-to-face oral examination. This shift in focus has resulted in a vast increase in the number of trials that include some form of either synchronous or asynchronous, teleconsultation/telediagnosis [18]. Thus, a successful translation of this technology into clinical practice has the ability to extend oral health care and improve access to care for additional patient populations at a reasonable cost, as well as to address the shortage of oral health professionals.

10.2.1 Improvements in the Quality of Services

In the case of residential aged care facility (RACF), by capturing video images locally, staff members avoid the disruption and difficulty of arranging transport for the residents to visit a dentist. There is anecdotal evidence from RACF staff that the stress imposed by travel to a dental surgery can lead to complete non-compliance with the dental examiner, to the point where attempts at oral examination are abandoned. This leads to further travel and reluctance on the part of patient and practitioner to repeat the process.

A timely diagnosis and follow-up appointment would improve quality of life of patients, as well as equity and access to expert dental care for patients living in regional areas; it can reduce the cost of treatment and the need to travel to urban centres to be seen by specialists, because dental problems can be identified via teledentistry. This reduces stress on residents and boosts their confidence that they are ‘in good hands’.

10.2.2 Improvements in the Quality of Care

The availability of high definition vision at the desktop enables a specialist clinician to use their time efficiently by reviewing data from multiple patients in one sitting, and prioritise appointments. For example, visiting domiciliary dentists will be aware of the exact nature of the problem before they arrive, this will result in time savings during treatment. They are able to plan a visit to treat the resident that coincides with other patients in the area, creating greater efficiency. The oral health professional will also be provided with better means of identifying older adults who require a diagnostic examination by a dental specialist.

Regarding specialist care, more patients can receive assessment and treatment, since patient care will be effectively triaged at the community level for subsequent care in a specialist centre. Thus, the approach would reduce waiting lists, a major problem in Australia due either to dental workforce shortages or its uneven geographic distribution. In addition, scarce resources are being utilised more efficiently.

10.2.3 Societal Perspective

Teledentistry can reduce health care inequalities, giving underserved communities better and fairer access to adequate oral health education, health promotion and disease prevention, diagnosis and treatment; as well as access to specialist dental services [5, 23]. People living in rural/remote or underserved areas are among the most in need of oral healthcare in their communities [2, 4]. Many rural/remote communities lack the clinical infrastructure and finances that are required to attract specialist dentists. Teledentistry can reduce the effect of remoteness by allowing oral healthcare providers in rural areas to seek advice from specialists in urban settings [2, 4].

An additional improvement from the patient's point of view arises from the greater convenience of being seen at a local dental clinic. Patients living in rural/remote areas who are referred to dental care providers in urban locations must travel to these locations which is often expensive, time consuming, and potentially stressful, particularly for the elderly. Teleconsultation helps general dental practitioners to consult with dental specialists for diagnosing a specific clinical condition, or to provide support for a colleague's clinical treatment decisions [9]. If an appropriate treatment plan can be devised prior to a direct patient-specialist visit, at least one preliminary appointment for the patient may be avoided [22].

From the health care system and societal perspective, the impact will be in the satisfaction of knowing that patients access appropriate care, and that scarce resources are being well utilized. In general, early intervention for dental problems reduces subsequent treatment costs and general health complications.

This also means that the high costs of patient stay at a hospital, and costs for numerous visits by the dentist have been avoided (note: in Australia adult dental care is not claimable under Medicare). Overall, teledentistry offers lower costs for higher quality care. Thus, the case for funding would be bolstered.

There are large potential savings for the health care system by allowing early intervention for dental problems by reducing the consequences of preventable oral health conditions (i.e. poor oral hygiene) such as dietary limitations and aspiration pneumonia amongst other chronic conditions. Substantial cost savings could also be made by minimising unnecessary journeys by specialist and support services. Public oral health care providers are short staffed and have long waiting lists. These savings would easily cover the cost of teledentistry implementations.

10.2.4 Digital Patient Recording and Record Repository

Associated patient data can be transferred simultaneously over the network connection. Data collected will be useful as a starting point for a large oral health record repository, which would combine digital records with periodontal and hard tissue charting, treatment notes, both moving and still images, and X-ray images. This combined patient record with searchable metadata would be stored in a central repository for further review, teaching and later dental health informatics research.

On the other hand, the implementation of these programs would create additional recurrent costs of maintaining the ICT equipment, such as cameras and laptops, as well as the central store and forward audio/video repository. These costs would need to be borne by an agency currently not bearing that cost. It could also create increased demand and pressures on existing dental services which may not be able to meet current demand. Teledentistry would also require workflow changes by dental specialists, which need to be taken into consideration.

In telehealth scenarios, various factors can affect data quality. Some of these may be anticipated and addressed, such as calibration of remote devices. Such issues may need to be elucidated before a wider implementation in which qualitative and human factors research, for instance, can highlight junctures where data quality, currency or timelag issues could be addressed. Digital data handling and management in teledentistry practice may additionally require renegotiation across stakeholders, depending on the source and intended purpose, format and expected longevity of the data [1, 12, 13].

10.3 Teledentistry 'Down Under'

Face-to-face patient examinations are regarded as the most accurate method for correct oral health diagnosis. However, rural and regional Australia has major oral health workforce shortages, in particular, oral health specialists (e.g., oral medicine, paediatric dentistry, maxillo-facial surgery). For example, to see a specialist, there is often a long waiting list for both consultation and treatment. Teledentistry seeks to provide and/or support oral health care in areas underserved by dental practitioners, transcending social, geographic, and cultural barriers [7]. This can also translate into reduced costs, improved patient outcomes and greater access to quality dental care [24].

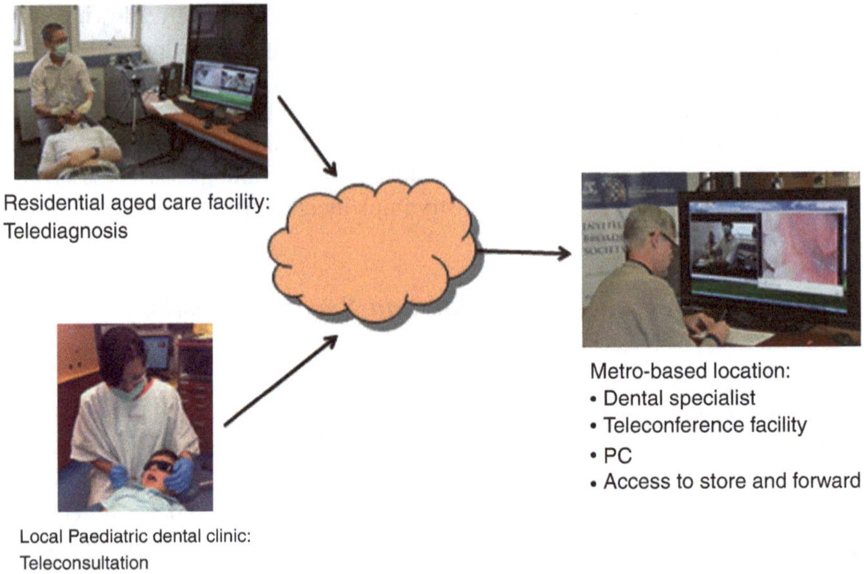

Fig. 10.1 Teledentistry installation diagram

This section presents results from three teledentistry projects: a proof-of concept study, a study targeting older adults living in residential care,[1] and another targeting children and adolescents living in regional and remote areas of the Australian state of Victoria. These studies investigated the use of teledentistry to provide an additional step in closing the gap in the provision of sustainable oral health care services to high-risk populations living in underserved areas, with extensive oral health care needs. The studies aimed to test an oral health model in which ICT was used with the objective of extending clinical care to patients who were physically separated from the examining oral health professional.

10.3.1 Proof-of-Concept of Teledentistry Technology

As a first stage a proof-of-concept study was undertaken to test the feasibility and reliability of using videoconference and intraoral cameras by a trained teledentistry assistant for screening of patients for oral diseases and conditions and development of treatment plans in real-time compared to traditional face-to-face oral examinations.

A teledentistry installation was organised using a SOPROLIFE®[2] intra-oral camera (Acteon, France) was used to capture video via a custom video streaming soft-

[1] A more detailed description of these studies can be found in: Mariño et al. [20].

[2] SOPROLIFE: Light Induced Fluorescence Evaluator. http://www.soprolife.com/. Accessed 23 Jan 2014.

ware platform designed for the project. Simulations were conducted in the Institute for Broadband Enabled Society (IBES http://broadband.unimelb.edu.au) test-bed facility. The intra-oral camera was connected via a USB cable to a laptop or mobile tablet used for bedside evaluations, containing the software that compressed and encoded the 25 frame-per-second video into an MP4 (Mpeg-4 multimedia file) video stream of a minimum of 3 Mbit/s data transfer rate – and preferably using 5 Mbit/s bandwidth if network conditions allowed (See Fig. 10.1). These bandwidths gave the clinician sufficient resolution quality to interpret the images received and also removed image blurring due to camera motion [19].

The clinician viewed the incoming video via a PC connected to a large monitor. The large screen facilitated simultaneous viewing of both the intra-oral camera video as well as that from a second web-cam, a high definition Logitech model C920 model, capturing the overall interaction between patient and the intra-oral camera operator. This was also streamed as an mpeg4 video of minimum 3 Mbit/s bandwidth. Mpeg4 audio was also transmitted at 128 kbit/s along with the images via the use of Clear One Chat 50 model microphone/speaker units also connected via USB cables. This allowed excellent quality audio communications between the patient and clinician nodes.

Fourteen volunteer patients received two oral examinations. One examination was a standard real-time (the clinician present in front of the patient) full mouth oral health examination including dental, periodontal and oral mucosal assessments. A second and 'virtual' examination was conducted using an intraoral camera operated by a teledentistry assistant in communication with a remote examiner who was also a registered oral health professional. The information obtained from this examination was video recorded and an oral health professional performed a 'virtual dental examination'. Findings were recorded in conventional dental charts.

Information from the remote examination was compared with a real-life dental examination. The level of intra-examination reliability for the degree of consistency of the two sets of examinations was assessed using the kappa statistic. The intra-examiner agreements for dental and periodontal examination parameters were reported as excellent, 0.94, and good, 0.74, respectively. These results indicate that the proposed teledentistry approach for oral health screening using an intraoral camera proved to be feasible and reliable as an alternative to traditional oral health examination.

10.3.2 Field Testing of Teledentistry Technology in Residential Aged Care Facilities

This study represented field testing of teledentistry technology to enhance older adult assessment in residential aged care facilities to provide regular and timely oral health checks using trained non-oral health professional assistants in the first instance. Improvements in oral health in Australia over the past 50 years have translated into a greater proportion of elderly individuals retaining more of their natural teeth, increasing the prevalence of caries and periodontal disease. Older people living in residential aged care facilities (RACFs) have been identified as a significant risk group for oral diseases in Australia, and the changing demography and oral health needs of older Australians will present many challenges for the dental profession over coming decades.

In 2005 more than 41,000 Victorians lived in high or low-care residential facilities on a permanent basis; with just over half being dentate and having high dental treatment needs [3, 15]. However in Victoria only 11 % of aged care facility residents have seen a dentist in the past 12 months, as there are few dentists available to provide dental care for residents [14, 16]. Furthermore, older people are proportionately over-represented in rural and regional Australian communities and these communities are ageing more rapidly than their metropolitan counterparts. Therefore, this intervention potentially targets a rapidly expanding segment of the population with special oral health needs.

Three RACFs within the state of Victoria, Australia, were successfully approached to participate in this stage; two in metropolitan Melbourne and one in rural Victoria. Five non-oral health professional teledental assistants (e.g., registered nurses) in these facilities were trained to manipulate an intraoral camera and use existing and introduced ICT infrastructure to transmit video images for remote examination and diagnosis. A manual was prepared to assist them with use of the intraoral camera and teledentistry procedures.

Once informed consent was provided, patients underwent a baseline assessment performed at the RACF, by the intraoral camera operator. A review system was established within the Melbourne Dental School, The University of Melbourne (MDS), either as a two-way interactive consultation, or stored and forwarded repository maintained by the MDS. A Store and Forward version was developed that enabled the mpeg4 file to be stored on a central server for asynchronous download by the dentists. Each examination lasted approximately 15 min and each minute of video created a file of approximately 1 GB.

Fifty residents from the three RACFs participated in the trial. A total of five trained intra-oral camera operators (registered nurses) recorded, and transmitted video images to qualified clinicians at the MDS who performed a 'virtual dental examination', recorded findings and developed a treatment plan for each participating resident. Results of the examination of each participating resident were communicated back to the RACF.

The study also aimed to identify barriers to the adoption of a teledental approach. On completing the virtual oral examination each participant was asked to complete a seven-item assessment questionnaire to assess his/her views on the teledentistry approach. As further verification of the scheme, there was an interview with the RACFs teledentistry staff to assess their attitude, acceptance and practice of the approach and to discuss any other issues encountered by them during the project. Residents expressed high levels of satisfaction with the teledentistry service.

Additionally, the trial tested the utility of an instructional training kit, and assessed residents' views of their overall experiences during delivery of the program, as well as feedback and information provided during the teledentistry consultation itself. There was general agreement that the material presented was clear and relevant to the purposes of this project. RNs also agreed that the scope of the material was appropriate.

10.3.3 Field Testing of Teledentistry for Paediatric Dentistry

The project targeted children and adolescents living in traditionally underserved regional and remote locations within the Australian state of Victoria to provide them with sustainable dental services. These are high-risk segments of the population with special oral health needs. The conjecture was that initial assessment by a consultant, using teledentistry, would decrease the number of times a patient would need to attend the Royal Children's Hospital in Melbourne (RCH) to see a specialist (i.e. orthodontist, paediatric dentist). In addition, the use of teleconsultation can help to categorise treatment priority and avoid the need for the patient to travel to an often distant centre for assessment.

In this study, three general dental practitioners (GDP) working in community dental clinics in Victoria (Rosebud, Shepparton, and Geelong) were trained to manipulate an intraoral camera and use existing ICT infrastructure to communicate with the dental specialist at RCH and transmit video images for remote examination. Training was provided for the GDP involved in the project and a manual was prepared to assist with use of the intraoral camera. A review system was established within the RCH as a two-way interactive consultation, almost equivalent to a real-time examination.

The trained GDP identified the reason for consultation, manipulated the intraoral camera and recorded findings for each participant. An off-site paediatric dentistry consultant located at the RCH, performed the 'virtual dental examinations'. The remote examiner screened patient and assessed their need for future intervention and provided advice on treatment to each participating patient and to the GDP and health staff at the local Community Health Centre. The remote examiner provided advice and follow-up to the GDP on how to manage the condition locally or refer for specialist care.

Participants were recruited from the RCH's patient database for cleft lip and palate (CL&P) and orthodontics living in the selected locations. Patients were introduced to the study by the GDP. When the patients, or their primary carers, expressed interest in participating, each received a Plain Language Statement describing the study and a Consent Form. Once informed consent was provided, patients underwent a baseline assessment. In common with the previous project, patients/parents of patients participating in the study completed a questionnaire to assess their experiences of the various aspects of the program; satisfaction, acceptance and practice of the teledentistry approach and to discuss issues associated with the project.

Forty-three remote assessments/consultations were conducted in two specific specialist service areas; 27 CL&P patients, and 15 in orthodontics. Additionally, one patient presented with Cohen's syndrome. Age ranged from 1 year and 11 months to 18 years of age. The largest group of patients (41.9 %) was between 4 and 8 years of age.

For most patients (82.9 %), the outcome of the consultation was the avoidance of trips to the centrally located RCH for initial assessment and/or follow-ups. Accordingly, approximately two-thirds of the parents who answered this question (75.6 %) commented that the most valuable element of the remote dental examination was the avoided disruption, difficulties and cost of arranging travel to the city to visit a dental specialist.

10.4 Outcomes

The major outcome was the trial of alternative models to provide specialist services to traditional oral health services provision in remote and underserved areas. The approaches provided general and specialist oral health care support to the local facilities to assist in regular and timely oral health checks using a GDP or trained non-oral health professional assistant in the first instance and specialist dental services when the required treatment was identified.

There was also evaluation of the support program and instruction kit for operators, including the structure, content and delivery of the program, as well as the relevance and appropriateness of the information provided. In summary, these field trails provided:

(i) initial evidence on how teledentistry might improve access to specialist care;
(ii) a pathway to improvements in the quality of care arising from consultant dental specialists being aware of the exact nature of the problem before the patient arrives;
(iii) identification of potential broader community benefits such as information on the level of convenience for both the family and the dental specialist; and
(iv) evidence of the generally excellent levels of acceptance of the virtual examination by patients and professionals working with children and the elderly.

10.5 Final Remarks

Building on these experiences, the next step will be the testing of an on-site oral health care model that can combine health promotion, remote oral examination and treatment plan development with a triage system, which can trigger different levels of clinical and preventive intervention by different oral health professionals (dental therapists/dental hygienists/technicians, dentists, dental specialists, etc.). As this will increase demand for local oral health care services, the proposed model will need to incorporate treatment opportunities to address the additional demand. For example, the remote examiner might provide advice to local health staff (or carer) on how to maintain the oral health of the participant, or provide advice to local private dentists with respect to the need for, and timing of, specialist care. Where these are not possible or available, and to avoid increased demand for local oral health care services, the proposed model would incorporate alternative service delivery systems to address the identified demand for dental care for older population groups in non-traditional settings.

Moreover, there are very few reports regarding the cost-effectiveness of teledentistry, so further studies in health economics are required before the widespread implementation of teledentistry into public health facilities, child-care centres, schools and clinical practices can be undertaken. The costs and benefits of proposed models should be measured to ensure that cogent arguments for future funding – utilising mechanisms that reflect the advantages accrued including service sustainability in the long-term – can be made to Government and philanthropic interests.

References

1. Ackerman MJ, Filart R, Poropatich RK. Developing next-generation telehealth tools and technologies: patients, systems, and data perspectives. Telemed J E Health. 2010;16:93–5.
2. Allukian M. The neglected epidemic and the surgeon general's report: a call to action for better oral health. Am J Public Health. 2008;98:S82–5.
3. Australian Institute of Health and Welfare. National Survey of Adult Oral Health 2004–2006. AIHW cat. no. DEN 165. Dental Statistics and Research Series No. 34; Canberra, Australian Institute of health and Welfare. 2008.
4. Beetstra S, Derksen D, Ro M, et al. A "health commons" approach to oral health for low-income populations in a rural state. Am J Public Health. 2008;98:S89–90.
5. Bradley M, Black P, Noble S, et al. Application of teledentistry in oral medicine in a community dental service, N. Ireland. Br Dent J. 2010;209:399–404.
6. Brüllmann D, Schmidtmann I, Warzecha K, et al. Recognition of root canal orifices at a distance – a preliminary study of teledentistry. J Telemed Telecare. 2011;17:154–7.
7. Chang SW, Plotkin DR, Mulligan R, et al. Teledentistry in rural California: a USC initiative. J Calif Dent Assoc. 2003;31:601–8.
8. Chen JW, Hobdell MH, Dunn K, et al. Teledentistry and its use in dental education. J Am Dent Assoc 2003;134:342–6.
9. Clark GT. Teledentistry: what is it now, and what will it be tomorrow? J Calif Dent Assoc. 2000;28:121–7.
10. Cook J, Austen G, Stephens C. Videoconferencing: what are the benefits for dental practice? Br Dent J. 2000;188:67–70.
11. Coulthard P, Kazakou I, Koran R, et al. Referral patterns and the referral system for oral surgery care. Part 2: the referral system and telemedicine. Br Dent J. 2000;188:388–91.
12. Davidson E, Simpson CR, Demiris G, et al. Integrating telehealth care-generated data with the family practice electronic medical record: qualitative exploration of the views of primary care staff. Interact J Med Res. 2013;2:e29. doi:10.2196/ijmr.2820.
13. Hanley J, Ure J, McKinstry B, et al. Self-care at home: user and carer's experiences of telemonitoring in the context of COPD, NIHR SDO and HSRN conference delivering better health services, 3–4 June 2009, Birmingham; 2009.
14. Hopcraft M, Morgan M, Satur J, et al. Dental service provision in Victorian residential aged care facilities. Aust Dent J. 2008;53:239–45.
15. Hopcraft M, Morgan M, Satur J, et al. Edentulism and dental caries in Victorian residential aged care facilities. Gerodontology. 2012;29:E512–9.
16. Hopcraft M, Morgan M, Satur J, et al. Oral hygiene and periodontal disease in Victorian residential aged care facilities. Gerodontology. 2012;29:220–8.

17. Kopycka-Kedzierawski DT, Billings RJ. Teledentistry in inner-city child-care centres. J Telemed Telecare. 2006;12:176–81.
18. Mariño R, Ghanim A. Teledentistry: a systematic review of the literature. J Telemed Telecare. 2013;19:189–94.
19. Mariño R, Hopcraft M, Collmann R, et al. A teledentistry approach for oral health screening in nursing homes. 2011. Available at: http://www.slideshare.net/ifa2012/3-mariooral-health-if-apresentation29may2012. Accessed 25 July 2014.
20. Mariño R, Marwaha P, Collmann R, Hopcraft M, Manton D, Stranieri A, Clarke K. Field testing of remote teledentistry technology. eTELEMED 2014: The Sixth International Conference on eHealth, Telemedicine, and Social Medicine.2014:23–28. Available at: http://www.thinkmind.org/index.php?view=article&articleid=etelemed_2014_2_10_40017. Accessed 25 July 2014.
21. Martin N, Lazalde OM, Stokes C, Romano D. An evaluation of remote communication versus face-to-face in clinical dental education. Br Dent J. 2012;212:277–82.
22. Sanchez Dils E, Lefebvre C, Abeyta K. Teledentistry in the United States: a new horizon of dental care. Int J Dent Hyg. 2004;2:161–4.
23. Scuffham PA, Steed M. An economic evaluation of the Highlands and Islands teledentistry project. J Telemed Telecare. 2002;8:165–77.
24. Sfikas PM. Teledentistry: legal and regularity issues explored. J Am Dent Assoc. 1997; 128:1716–8.

Index

A

Access to oral care
- advocacy and policy change, 73
- categorical demographic variables, 72
- CD, 72
- clinical screening intraoral images, 71
- dental caries, 66–68
- dental hygienists, 70–71
- dental insurance, 68
- dental professionals, 69
- dentition and early care, 68
- electronic radiographs and health record, 72
- health-care disparities and barriers, 69
- mobile equipment, 71
- PPACA, 69
- retractors and intraoral mirrors, 71
- rural and urban areas, 68
- Wilcoxon Sign Ranks test, 72

Adaptive devices, 36, 39

Alaska Dental Health Aide Therapist (DHAT), 61

Alaska Federal Health Care Access Network (AFHCAN), 61

AM. *See* Antemortem (AM)

American Recovery and Reinvestment Act (ARRA), 2

Antemortem (AM)
- 3D craniofacial reconstruction, 79
- dentists, 78
- extra-and intraoral photographs, 76

Australia, teleconsultation and telediagnosis
- application, 102
- benefits, 103–105
- digital patient recording and record repository, 104–105
- face-to-face patient examinations, 105
- field testing
  - paediatric dentistry, 108–110
  - residential aged care facilities, 107–109
- ICT, 102
- installation diagram, 106
- outcomes, 110
- paediatric dentistry, 109–110
- proof-of-concept, 106–107
- quality of care, 104
- quality of services, 103
- RACFs, 107–109
- societal perspective, 104–105

B

BigMouth (large dental data repository), 9

Bitemark analysis
- antemortem/postmortem, 80, 81
- dental alignments, size, shape and dental arches, 80, 81
- face, stomach and buttocks, 80
- technologies, 81–82

Brazilian Association of Dental Education, 91

Brazilian Telehealth Program, 89, 92

Brazil, teledentistry
- Centers of Dental Specialties, 89
- Dental Telepropaedeutics, 92
- distance-learning courses, 91
- educational policy, guidelines, 88
- eHealth as national policy, 88
- eHealth strategies, 89
- Family Health Teams, 89
- geographic problems, 92
- human health resources, 88
- ICT, benefits, 93

S. Kumar (ed.), *Teledentistry*, Health Informatics,
DOI 10.1007/978-3-319-08973-7

Brazil, teledentistry (*cont.*)
interactive teleducation, 87
Millenium Development Goals (MDG), 88
National Teledentistry Network–RNTO, 89
Teledentistry Centre FOUSP School of Dentistry, University of São Paulo, 94–98
Telemedicine, Department of FMUSP, 91
Virtual Human (project), 91, 96

C
Caries
assessment methods
detection methods, 26
fluorescence-based detection systems, 30–32
optical scattering detection systems, 26–30
oral health care benefit, 23
teledentistry, 24
TLS (*see* Teledentistry lesion scale (TLS))
caregivers, 67
children, 67
detection methods, 26
DFS, 66
DFT score, 66
management, 24
pain, 67
SES, 66
CBCT. *See* Cone-beam computed tomography (CBCT)
CD. *See* Clinical dentist (CD)
Charged couple device (CCD), 77
Cleft lip and palate (CL&P), 109
Clinical dentist (CD), 50, 71, 72, 94
Cloud-based EHR, 10
CL&P. *See* Cleft lip and palate (CL&P)
Cone-beam computed tomography (CBCT), 78
Confidentiality, 5–6
Congress of Brazilian Council for Telemedicine and Telehealth (CBTms), 93
Cross-polarization optical coherence tomography (CP-OCT)
diagnosis, 29
and MID, 27
scorings, 28

D
Data repository, 9
Daubert guidelines, 84
3D computerized reconstructions, 79
Decayed and filled primary teeth (DFT) scores, 66
Decayed and filled surfaces (DFS), 66, 70, 72
Dental health education, 38
Dental hygienists
Apple Tree model, 61
Arizona's affiliated practice, 44
clinical dentist (CD), 72
dental chart, 71
ECC and S-ECC, 70
intraoral imagess, 70
licensed dentists, 69
methodology, 71
NAU, 45–46
occupational therapist, 39
oral cavity, 70
oral healthcare services, 43
skills and knowledge, 69
teledentisty equipment, 60
Digital imaging and communications in medicine (DICOM), 49, 50, 77
Doctor-patient relationship
computer and monitor positioning, 4
computer, dental operatory, 4
ethics, 6–7
health information, 5
monitor and/ all-in-one computer placement, 4, 5
privacy, security and confidentiality issues, 5–6

E
Early childhood caries (ECC), 70
Electronic health records (EHRs)
advantages, 2
ARRA, 2
clinician, 8
cloud-based, 10
COHRI project, 9
computers, 2–3
data repository, 9
dental, 55–56
description, 1–2
doctor-patient relationship (*see* Doctor-patient relationship)
ethics, 6–7
HIE, 55
HITECH Act, 54
implementation, 2
interconnectivity, 3
practitioners, 7–8
re-using, 8
security and confidentiality, health information, 5–6
SNODENT, 54–55

F
Federal Council of Dentistry (CFO), 95
Federal University of Paraná (UFPR), 93
Federal University of Rio Grande do Sul–UFRGS, 91
Fluorescence-based detection systems
  dentinal caries, 31–32
  signal, 30–31
  teledentistry, 31
Forensic odontology
  accidental and nonaccidental injuries, 82–83
  bitemarkanalysis, 80–82
  CBCT, 78
  CT, MRI and surface scanning, 78–79
  digital dental records and radiography
    burn victim identification, 77
    clear cementoenamel junction, 77
    description, 76
    PM, 76–77
    scanning electron microscopy, 77
    x-ray fluorescence spectrometer (XRF), 77, 78
  digital photography, 76
  medico-legal implications, 84
  MFI, 75–76
  RFID tag, 79
  software and databases, 80
  three-dimensional craniofacial reconstruction, 79

G
General dental practitioners (GDP), 14, 15, 104, 109, 110
Geriatric dentistry, 97
Global positioning system (GPS), 76

H
Health information exchange (HIE), 55
Health Information Technology for Economic and Clinical Health (HITECH) Act, 2, 6, 54
Health Insurance Portability and Accountability Act (HIPAA), 6, 7, 9, 54
Health on the Net Foundation (HON), 94
Home telecare
  cognitive impairment/physical disabilities, 37–38
  concept, 36
  definition, 35
  description, 35
  evolution, 36
  health care professionals, 38–39
  members/providers, 39–40
  OHTQ, 37
  oral hygiene behaviors, 36

I
Information and communication technologies (ICT), 88, 89, 93, 94, 98, 102, 103, 105, 106, 108, 109
Interactive teleeducation, 87
International Classification of Diseases (ICD), 92
International Open Access movement, 98
Intra-oral camera
  blurred image, 49
  color monitor, 15
  disposable sheath barriers, 51
  GDP, 109
  KinderCamp Head Start project, 50
  logitech model, 107
  mouth mirror, 49
  non-oral health professional teledental assistants, 108
  prototype, 18
  teledentistry, 24
  videoconference, 106
  visual oral health screen, 14
  x-ray mannequin, 47

M
Mass fatality incident (MFI), 75–76, 78
Medical records, 50, 54
Medicolegal identifications, 41, 75. *See also* Forensic odontology

N
NACOG. *See* Northern Arizona Council of Governments (NACOG)
National Coordination for the Improvement of Higher Education of the Ministry of Education (CAPES/MEC), 98
National Teledentistry Network–RNTO, 89, 91, 96
National Telehealth Program, 91, 96
Northern Arizona Council of Governments (NACOG), 50–51
Northern Arizona University (NAU)
  classroom presentation, 50
  dental hygiene, 45–46
  DICOM, 49
  training endeavors, 45
  training methods and materials, 47
  x-ray scanning device, 48–49

O

OHTQ. *See* Oral home telecare questionnaire (OHTQ)
Open University of the Unified National Health System–UNA SUS, 89, 97
Optical scattering detection systems, 26–30
Oralcare
  education and training, 39
  outcomes, 55
Oral health assessment
  health economics, 111
  ICT, 102
  informatics, 103
  program and instruction kit, 110
  teledentistry, 103–110
  telemedicine, 102
  triage system, 110
Oral home telecare questionnaire (OHTQ), 37
Oral manifestations, 18–19
Oral medicine
  concept, 14
  management, 14
  teledentistry, 17
  telehealth, 14
Oral mucosal disease
  consultants, 17
  digital images and clinical details, 15–16
  medicine, 14, 17
  oral maxillofacial surgery, 14
  preliminar appraisal, 18–19
  prototype teledentistry system, 18
  teleconsultations, 15
  teledentistry, 14
  telehealth, 14, 20
  "telemedicine rounds," 18
  temporomandibular joint disorders, 14

P

Paediatric dentistry, 91, 94, 95, 97, 105, 109–110
Pan American Health Organization (PAHO), 91, 97
Patient Protection and Affordable Care Act (PPACA), 45, 69
Periodontal examination, 107
Plain Language Statement, 109
Postmortem (PM)
  CBCT, 78
  dental records, 76
  odontological method, 78

R

Radio frequency identification tags (RFID tag), 79
Registered dental assistants (RDA), 61
Registered dental hygienists (RDH), 61
Registered dental hygienists in alternative practice (RDHAP), 61
Remote monitoring method, 57
Residential aged care facility (RACFs), 103, 107–109
RFID tag. *See* Radio frequency identification tags (RFID tag)
Root-transparency level, 80
Royal Children's Hospital in Melbourne (RCH), 109, 110

S

S-ECC. *See* Severe early childhood caries (S-ECC)
Security, EHR. *See* Electronic health records (EHRs)
Severe early childhood caries (S-ECC), 70
Systemized Nomenclature of Dentistry (SNODENTr), 54–55

T

Technology
  computer, 49
  DICOM, 50
  telecommunication, 57
  telehealth, 53
Teledentistry and dental hygiene
  advantages, 58–60
  DHAT and AFHCAN, 61
  disadvantages, 60–61
  EHRs (*see* Electronic health records (EHRs))
  federal government, 53
  history, 56–57
  RDH and RDA, 61
  RDHAP, 61
  real-time consultation and store-and-forward, 57, 58
  remote monitoring method, 57
  technological requirements, 57–59
  telehealth, 53
Teledentistry Centre FOUSP School of Dentistry, University of São Paulo
  APS–VHL (Virtual Health Library in Primary Care), 97

asynchronous and synchronous communication tools, 94
Centre for Teledentistry FOUSP, 94
Centres for Telehealth and Teledentistry, 94–95
Current Profile and Trends of the Brazilian Dental Surgeon (project), 95
digital content, activities, 95
Endodontic Technique FOUSP, 94
Geriatric dentistry, ODL course, 97
Integration with Telehealth Programs, 98
National Network Teledentistry, 98
Open University of SUS (UNA-SUS), 96
Primary Care Dental Health, 95
second opinions, oral health topics, 97
technological innovations, use of, 94
training program, Department of Paediatric Dentistry, 95
Teledentistry lesion scale (TLS), 24–25
Telehealth
information technology, 18
in oral medicine, 14–15
technologies, 53
tools, 91
Telehealth Centers of the University of the State of Rio de Janeiro–UERJ, 91
Telemedicine University Network–RUTE, 89
Telerehabilitation, 39
TLS. *See* Teledentistry lesion scale (TLS)
Training materials, teledentistry, 46–50
Training methodologies, NAU. *See* Northern Arizona University (NAU)

U

Unified Health System (SUS), 88
Unified Victim Identification System (UVIS), 80
UVIS Dental Identification Module (UVIS/UDIM), 80

V

Video conferencing, 59, 60
Virtual Human (project), 91, 96

X

X-ray fluorescence spectrometer (XRF), 77, 78